REHAB YOUR OWN

Spinal Stenosis

REHAB YOUR OWN

REHAB YOUR OWN

SPINAL STENOSIS
Strategies to Improve the Health of Your Spine

Terri Night, M.S.P.T.

To Esther Draznin,
role model and friend

Table of Contents

Published by Terrific Books
ISBN-13 978-1732264205
ISBN-10 1732264201

www.rehabspinalstenosis.com

Book Design by John Hubbard / EMKS.fi
Illustrations by Tim McGee (unless otherwise credited)
Cover photo of author by Ahamed Iqbal
Cover design by Karla Hernandez and John Hubbard

DISCLAIMER

The material contained in these pages is not a substitute for medical evaluation and diagnosis by a physician. Nor is this material a substitute for the kind of fine-tuning and personalized treatment you would get from a good physical therapist. However, if physical therapy has failed to help you in the past, you may find strategies in this book that work. Reading this book prior to starting any type of treatment will make you a more knowledgeable and prepared collaborator with your chosen healthcare practitioner.

If you have symptoms of spinal stenosis and have not been evaluated by a medical doctor, please do so. Always consult a physician before beginning any new exercise program or treatment plan.

The cases presented in this book are based on my 28 years of experience as a licensed physical therapist, but none of them represents an actual case. The individuals described are composites created to enhance understanding and to ensure anonymity.

To protect the identities of those involved, I have
altered certain details of individual case studies.

Introduction

INTRODUCTION

SUCCESS STORIES

BUD, 60-year-old retired construction worker

MRI RESULT:

*"Severe central canal stenosis related
to a large disc protrusion at L5-S1"*

Bud struggled with a strange, heavy—almost cramping—feeling in his legs and low back after walking more than 10 minutes. He also felt like he was developing a stoop.

Within one month of rehabbing his own spinal stenosis, Bud's symptoms completely resolved and he returned to daily 45-minute walks.

LORRAINE, 74-year-old retired dentist

MRI RESULT:

"Severe spondylolisthesis at L3-4 and L4-5 with narrowing of the spinal canal and pressure on the spinal cord and nerve root."

Lorraine had severe constant pain in her low back and hips. She was unable to turn in bed comfortably, and had difficulty getting up from a chair. Lorraine used to walk for an hour every day, but now she could barely walk across the house. Her pain, tingling, and weakness moved from the front of her thighs, to the back of her thighs, to one or both calves.

Within two months of rehabbing her own spinal stenosis, Lorraine's symptoms were 90% resolved. She returned to her daily walking routine.

MRI RESULT:

"Mild spondylolisthesis at L5-S1 with severe bony spurring in the lateral L4-5 nerve canal with direct pressure on the nerve root."

Yukio had constant burning in his low back that ran down the front of his right thigh. He used a cane and leaned forward and away from the right side as he limped along. Yukio couldn't even walk to the bathroom without severe pain. "The funny thing is, it goes away as soon as I sit down."

Within six months of rehabbing his own spinal stenosis, Yukio was riding his bike symptom-free for an hour a day, walking without a limp or a cane, and was no longer stooped over. He also enrolled in an industrial re-training program.

MRI RESULT:

"Severe spinal stenosis, osteoporosis, and compression fractures."

Sylvia had constant burning in her low back and a terrible time sleeping. She hunched way over when she walked, her knees buckling a little with each step, and grabbed walls and furniture to make her way across the room. "I can't even stand up long enough to cook dinner." Although afraid of falling, Sylvia refused to use a walker, since "the next step from there is straight into a nursing home!"

Within one month of rehabbing her own spinal stenosis, Sylvia could sleep through the night and felt 50% better. Within two months of rehabbing her own spinal stenosis she was able to cook for herself easily and take 15-minute daily walks. She still walked bent over a little, but no longer used walls or furniture to get across the room.

The above individuals come from different walks of life, but they all have the following things in common:

- They all had severe spinal stenosis shown on an MRI.
- They all successfully rehabbed their own spinal stenosis.
- They all did it *without having surgery*.

These profiles are based on clients of mine--clients who taught me one of my most valuable lessons: Using the same basic principles I've been teaching for years, even people with severe stenosis can improve their symptoms dramatically.

I'm here to tell you that you can too!

THE STENOSIS DIAGNOSIS

Spinal stenosis (a narrowing of the spinal canal or of the nerve openings in the spine) is most common in people over 50. If you're over 60, you have a 50% chance of having some degree of spinal stenosis. Since people over 60 account for 11% of the population, that's a lot of narrowed nerve openings and spinal canals!

Just hearing the words *spinal stenosis* can have a depressing effect. If it's this difficult to pronounce, it must be bad, right? Recently diagnosed people often picture worst-case scenarios:

>*Am I going to be paralyzed?*

>*I'm afraid I'll wind up in a wheelchair...*

>*The only thing that's going to fix this is surgery, right?*

For most people with stenosis, the answers to the above are: No. No. And definitely not.

Hopefully, the information I'm about to give you will help. Many people with spinal stenosis are living symptom-free, and many more are living with only minimal discomfort. A 2006 study of *symptom-free* people over the age of 55 found that 6% of them unknowingly had severe spinal stenosis. Can you believe it? These are people who didn't even know they had stenosis and weren't doing anything at all to manage it consciously!

Of course, those are just some numbers on people without symptoms. What about those of you who are already suffering? Didn't Bud, Lorraine, Yukio, and Sylvia make rather exceptional improvements? Yes, they did. But they are not alone. I've seen these types of improvements many times with clients—it never stops surprising me what the human body can do.

A Quick Note on Surgery

Of course, I don't want to discourage the person who really needs surgery. If you have a severe neurological deficit, you may not have much choice. Back surgery techniques have come a long way toward minimizing complications and improving recovery times. If you are about to have (or have already had) surgery for spinal stenosis, *Rehab Your Own Spinal Stenosis* will grease the wheels for your best possible recovery. Why? Because the same things that lead to a healthy spine in folks who don't need surgery lead to a healthy spine in folks who need it or have had it.

That being said, I must admit I *do* have a little bit of a bias. Unlike something like acute appendicitis, spinal stenosis is typically not a rapidly progressing problem. Waiting several years to have surgery has no effect on the ultimate outcome or prognosis. This waiting can be to your benefit. Consider this:

- *Spinal stenosis surgery puts you at risk for complications*. To list a few: wound infection, bladder infection, dural tears, stroke, heart attack, anesthesia- induced mental fog, and irreversible nerve damage.
- *Spinal stenosis symptoms can improve without surgery*. These improvements occur at every level of stenosis, from mild to severe.

This is why spine surgeons often refer stenosis patients to physical therapy first. It just makes good sense. It makes me think of a sign I saw posted at one of the check-out lanes in the grocery store the other day. The sign said:

PLEASE ALLOW US TO SERVE YOU
AT ONE OF THE OTHER REGISTERS.

When I finished reading, I found myself smiling. What a fabulously genteel alternative to the old-fashioned:

THIS REGISTER IS CLOSED.

Please allow us to serve you at one of the other registers... Regarding back surgery, my message is:

PLEASE ALLOW ME TO SERVE YOU WITH
ONE OF THE OTHER OPTIONS.

That option would be—again for *many* of you, not all—the non-surgical option. It may be hard to believe, but your surgeon prefers it too.

Spinal stenosis is not your ordinary back pain. In fact, it is quite different. And some instructions for ordinary back pain can make spinal stenosis worse. Hence, being on the receiving end of a lot of well-meaning "friendly" advice can be a real pain in the butt. And I mean this literally. One of the reasons I wrote this book was to give people the tools to ward off misguided advice, to clear the murky waters of Is this good or bad for me? In these pages, you'll find answers to questions like:

How did this spinal stenosis thing happen to a nice person like me?

Why am I always hunching forward?

Should I force myself to stand up straight?

If my spinal canal is narrowed, how is exercise going to change that?

Is there one specific muscle I can strengthen to cure this?

Rehab Your Own Spinal Stenosis explains what spinal stenosis is and how or why it may affect you. I'll reveal how you—just like Bud, Lorraine, Yukio, and Sylvia— can optimize the chances of being symptom-free using a variety of tools, including:

- A Personalized Exercise Program
- Strategies to Minimize Pressure on the Spinal Cord and Nerves
- Specialized Equipment
- Improvements in Wellness

As a physical therapist, I've been working with spinal stenosis patients for over 25 years, keeping track of the latest research and collaborating with thousands to develop their home rehab programs. Most are surprised to find out there are many ways to relieve their symptoms, simple do-it-yourself tricks I'll share with you to put you back in control. Although not every piece of advice or exercise in this book applies to your situation, you'll be able to find more than a few that will. Ultimately, you'll come away with a better understanding of why your symptoms may come and go, and how dealing with stenosis is less about "fixing" the problem and more about managing it better. When your stenosis is managed in the best possible way, your overall quality of life improves.

Five years ago, I sat across from an angry client who thought her doctor "dumped" her in physical therapy because he didn't know what else to do. At the end of our first session, her eyes welled-up with tears. "Why didn't anyone tell me this stuff before?"

That day, I went home and decided to write *this stuff* down.

Maybe you've been recently diagnosed. Maybe you've lived with spinal stenosis for years. Maybe you've already had surgery and want to avoid another one. Maybe you only have mild spinal stenosis and want to keep it that way. Maybe you have moderate or severe stenosis and feel like surgery is your only option. Whatever your situation, I wrote *Rehab Your Own Spinal Stenosis* to teach you everything I know, so that you can be a more knowledgeable and prepared collaborator with your chosen healthcare provider.

So, without further ado...

**PLEASE ALLOW ME TO SERVE YOU WITH
ONE OF THE OTHER OPTIONS.**

REHAB YOUR OWN: SPINAL STENOSIS
IS DIVIDED INTO THREE PARTS:

PART ONE: *The Stenosis Diagnosis*, explains spinal stenosis and, of course, includes a little bit of anatomy and physiology. I try to demystify the diagnosis, without getting too mired down in boring medical terms and details. (My favorite thing about writing this section is that I figured out how to make a model of the lumbar spine using nothing but toothpicks, glazed donuts, Oreo cookies, and a licorice rope.). You will learn that stenosis is a combination of many different factors—some of them impossible to change, and some of them very easy. In the end, you'll be able to better visualize how the approaches in Part Two work.

PART TWO: *Three Focus Areas*, details the main focus areas you can use to manage your stenosis:

- FOCUS AREA 1: *Decrease Inflammation*
  Learn why I consider inflammation to be the "X" factor in the battle against spinal stenosis symptoms. I'll talk about how swelling not only takes up space in the spine, but weakens muscles that support the spine. You'll come away with several different approaches to reducing inflammation.

- FOCUS AREA 2: *Keep Moving with Strategic Exercise*
  The goal of this section is to shift the view of exercise as *strengthening only* to the view of exercise as *improving circulation, decreasing inflammation, and correcting faulty movement patterns*. You'll be able to choose from a number of simple non-aggravating exercises described and diagrammed. (Videos of the exercises in greater detail are also available on my website.) I'll discuss some easy-to-use exercise equipment, motivational strategies, and how to plan a walking program.

- FOCUS AREA 3: *Improve Health and Wellness*
  Discover the role of wellness in relation to spinal stenosis and explore various areas of wellness you may need to address.

PART THREE: *Surgery*, gives definitions of some surgical terms, and describes what to expect after an operation for stenosis. (There, you see? I'm not *totally* anti-surgery.) You will also get some advice on important screening questions for a potential spine surgeon.

Finally, there's an *Appendix* with a list of "25 Handy Tips for Lumbar Spinal Stenosis" and a "Glossary of Terms."

PART ONE

The Stenosis Diagnosis

TAKING THE FIRST STEP

The most important step in rehabbing your own spinal stenosis? First, make sure you *have* spinal stenosis. To do this, you need to see a physician. There may be other more serious causes for your symptoms, and it's important to rule those out.

The following pages will help explain your diagnosis. They are not intended to help you diagnose yourself.

WHAT IS SPINAL STENOSIS?

The word *stenosis* is defined as an abnormal narrowing of any opening in the body. You can have *aortic valve stenosis* (narrowing at the valve to the major artery of the heart), *bronchial stenosis* (narrowing of the bronchial tube of the lung), or *intestinal stenosis*, which is, well, just...very unpleasant. The term *spinal stenosis* relates to an abnormal narrowing of either the spinal cord canal or of the nerve openings. Think of a piece of Swiss cheese. Swiss cheese has holes big enough for spinal nerves to pass through. Change that cheese to a baby Swiss, suddenly the holes aren't big enough—and, it's kind of like this in your spine.

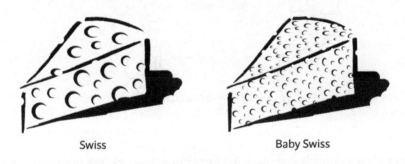

Swiss   Baby Swiss

(This is not meant in any way to disparage baby Swiss cheese,
which is a fine cheese for sandwiches or even just a snack.)

When the holes in the spine are narrowed like this, people can experience:

- severe low back pain
- feelings of heaviness or pressure in the low back
- weakness or cramping in the legs
- difficulty standing up straight (pain eased by bending forward)
- loss of balance
- pain or weakness relieved by sitting
- pain and weakness increasing with prolonged standing
- (in severe cases) loss of bowel or bladder function

CRASH COURSE ANATOMY

There are 33 bones in the human spine: 24 separated by discs, 9 fused. The fused bones are at the very base of the spine and make up your sacrum and tailbone.

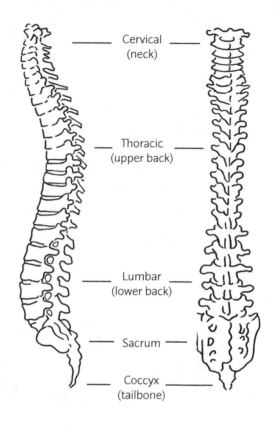

Cervical (neck)

Thoracic (upper back)

Lumbar (lower back)

Sacrum

Coccyx (tailbone)

You can have stenosis any place in your spine: the neck, the mid-back, or low back—but the low back accounts for 75% of cases. For simplicity's sake, this book deals only with spinal stenosis in your low back area—or lumbar spinal stenosis.

Here's a view of the lumbar spine:

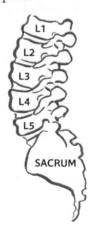

L1
L2
L3
L4
L5
SACRUM

As you can see, the bones are numbered 1 through 5, with an "L" in front that stands for lumbar. Below those five lumbar spine bones, you can also see the sacrum, which looks, from the side, like a little inverted powder horn. Or a pork chop.

TWO TYPES OF SPINAL STENOSIS

There are two types of spinal stenosis: central canal stenosis and foraminal stenosis. In laymen's terms, central canal means the hole down the middle (for the spinal cord) and foraminal refers to the holes on the sides (for the nerves). Think about a donut. In a way, each individual bone in your spine is like a donut. Not fluffy. Not delicious. But with a big round hole in the middle.

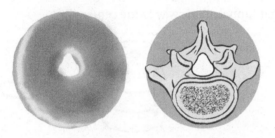

If you decided to stack 24 Krispy Kremes on top of each other, you'd have a long tunnel right down the middle:

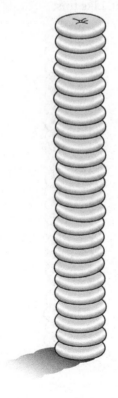

If these stacked donuts were actually the bones of a human spine, the hole down the middle is what the spinal cord runs through.

Central stenosis

When there is pressure on your spinal cord—as can happen when the hole down the middle narrows (central stenosis)—pain, cramping, and weakness, as well as numbness and tingling, may travel down both your legs at the same time.

Foraminal Stenosis

Let's imagine that stack of donuts again. I'm going to take a knife and start cutting holes in it, holes that tunnel all the way to the center.

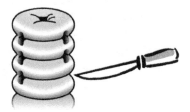

I keep cutting these holes until I have one on either side, taking up part of the upper and lower part of each donut. Like this:

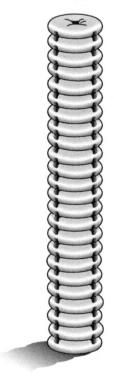

In the human spine, this would be where the nerves come out.

When there is pressure on your spinal nerve, as can happen when one of the holes on the side narrows (foraminal stenosis) let's say on the right side of your lumbar spine, then you will probably feel it on your right side. It may be a burning pain down the back of your right leg or feel like a hot poker being driven into your right butt cheek. (Ouch, right?) Many people have narrowed holes on both sides and get a dose of misery in both legs. Some have worse narrowing on one side and have pain down the opposite leg—what would seem to be the wrong leg. And others have narrowing of all three holes—and have no pain or weakness at all. Go figure. This is an illustration of how every human is different—and how what you see on your MRI or CT scan may not correspond exactly to what you feel.

WHAT CAUSES NARROWING OF THE SPINAL CANAL AND NERVE OPENINGS?

Clients often ask me: "So, what's causing all this narrowing?" That's when I pull out my plastic model of the spine and give them a laundry list of possibilities:

- bony changes
- bulging or collapsed discs
- enlarged, thickened, or loosened ligaments
- changes in connective tissue (fascia)
- swelling

Some of the above are a natural part of aging (though they can be congenital—in which case someone quite young could have spinal stenosis), and some are caused by wear and tear. Some are caused by what you do during the day, and how you use your body habitually. In fact, with most spinal stenosis, it is not one particular element that is responsible for everything, but a combination of several. I will discuss each in order to give you a better understanding of the whole.

> Note: The space available for your spinal cord and nerves is always changing. It changes depending on what time of day it is. It changes depending on what position you're in. It changes with certain movements. And it changes depending on the amount of load or pressure you've put on your spine.

Bony Changes

If you do heavy work in the garden you get calluses (build-up of skin) on your hands. If you do heavy work in your life, you get calluses (build-up of bone) on your spine bones. The bones in your spine (or vertebrae) change shape as you age. Sometimes, they collapse in on themselves:

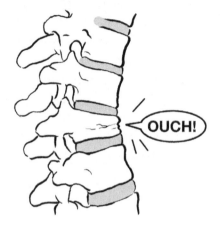

And sometimes, they develop spurs (bony projections, also called osteophytes). Spurs often poke out in unfortunate directions:

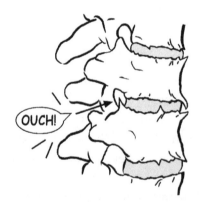

Some are shaped like little parakeet beaks!

Some spurs won't cause you any trouble at all. In the above drawing, though, you can see one spur jutting right into the space where the nerve would come out. As my realtor likes to say, "It's all about location. Location, location, location!" And that's definitely a bad location for a spur!

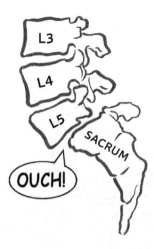

Sometimes one spine bone slips forward on the other because of a tiny fracture.

This slippage is known as *spondylolisthesis*.

Is it possible to change the bones in your spine? Well, in some ways, yes. And in other ways, no. Can you undo spondylolisthesis, a spur, or a collapse? No, not really. Can you prevent them from getting worse—or at least slow the deterioration? Yes. Since spurs form as a result of spinal instability, strengthening the muscles that stabilize the spine can slow the growth of spurs. In addition, increasing the flow of blood and nutrients to your spine (via exercise, nutrition, and wellness changes) will make your bones much healthier overall.

Bulging or Collapsed Discs

Twenty-four of the bones in your spine are separated by discs. Discs act as shock absorbers and create space between the spine bones to facilitate movement. They also flatten out naturally over time. If you traumatize your spine (like with a football injury or a car accident), that whole flattening thing can happen even faster. Ever watched a retired professional football linebacker walk?

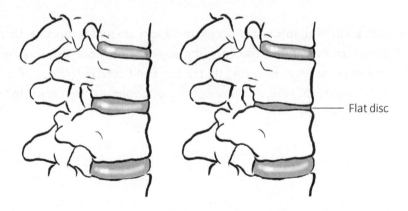

Flat disc

27

Calluses also can form on the discs, making them bulge or protrude out toward the spinal cord. Sometimes this is just an old injury to the disc that's gotten bigger and bigger over time.

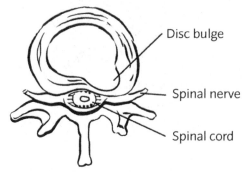

Disc bulge

Spinal nerve

Spinal cord

What's the difference between a "slipped disc," a "bulging disc" and a "disc protrusion"? Why, not a thing. They are the same.

What's the difference between the disc of a 20-year-old and the disc of a 55- or 60-year-old? How about the difference between the disc of a 30-year-old and a 70-year-old? Using types of food can be a fun way to compare!

20–year-old disc: *jelly donut*

30–year-old disc: *fresh crab*

40–year-old disc: *imitation crab*

50–year-old disc: *steak—medium*

60–year-old disc: *steak—well done*

70–year-old disc: *beef jerky*

90–year-old disc: *a shriveled hint of what was
once something like beef jerky*

100–year-old disc: *"I have a disc?"*

The main point of all this is that people of all ages are told by doctors, therapists, and chiropractors that their discs are like jelly donuts. These poor souls go around all spinal steno-stressed, worrying that if they bend over, the jelly-stuff in their discs will "squirt out." Well, if you're 65 years old, your disc isn't going to "squirt" out anything. You can relax.

Still, the health of a single disc can play a large part in spinal stenosis.

- **It can bulge out into the *spinal canal* (spinal cord hole) or *foramina* (nerve exit-hole).** That wayward bit of disc can put direct pressure on your nerve or spinal cord. Or it can rub against structures like bones, tendons, or ligaments —creating friction, irritation, and swelling.
- **It can become so flat the vertebrae aren't separated enough to move properly.** Edges of bone grind against ligaments, tendons, and whatever's left of your disc (they even grind against each other!) creating—you guessed it—friction, irritation, and swelling. All this adds up to less room for the spinal cord. Decreased cord space! It also adds up to smaller nerve canals—less room for your nerves!

Many times, a single disc can have both problems. A flattened-out disc can easily be a sticking-out disc too.

Is it possible to change the discs in your spine? Indeed it is. In fact, you can do it even from moment to moment! This is because your discs are changing from moment to moment anyway! The height of a disc (which has to do with its hydration level) varies depending on what time of day it is, how long you've been sitting, and even how much load you're carrying.

TRUE OR FALSE?
The height of your discs as shown on an MRI can be affected by how long you sat in the waiting room?

ANSWER:
True.

Another piece of good news: Discs do have a blood supply. Why is that good news? Because you can control the blood supply to your discs! What? How can I do that? Well, it's amazingly easy. All you have to do is exercise. It doesn't even matter what type of exercise you do. As long as you do it long enough to increase circulation. How long is long enough? Check this out! Even a good 10-minute warm-up can increase the number of open capillary beds in a particular area by as much as 100 times.

The blood supply to the discs is responsible for:

- providing nutrition to disc cells
- providing hydration to the disc

If you improve nutrition to your discs, the disc cells become healthier and more resilient. The fluid content of a disc is not constant, but varies throughout the day depending position, activity, and load. If you improve disc hydration, your disc becomes less flat. This creates more space between your bones so they can move without bumping up against each other and all creation. See how the nerve opening is much smaller when the disc is flat?

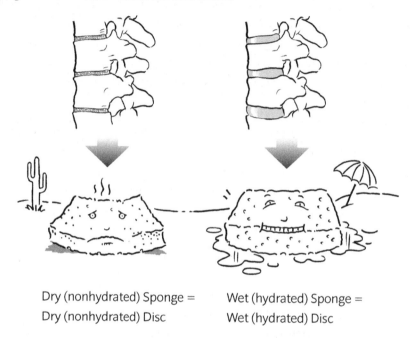

Dry (nonhydrated) Sponge =
Dry (nonhydrated) Disc

Wet (hydrated) Sponge =
Wet (hydrated) Disc

Hence, any exercise that's good for your circulatory system is also good for your discs. And if you can improve the health of your discs, you can increase the space for your spinal cord and nerves. Simply by exercising to improve circulation, you can—and likely will—reduce symptoms of spinal stenosis.

Enlarged Thickened or Loosened Ligaments

Ligaments are like belts and ropes, the cinches of human tissue. They connect bones to other bones, and basically hold things together. Healthy ligaments are elastic, lengthening under tension, and returning to their original shape when tension is removed. Ligaments that lose their elasticity are like old rubber bands put on slack. They just wad up and take up space.

Two major ligaments live *inside* the spinal canal. One long ligament lines the front of the canal, and the other (which is actually a series of small ligaments) lines the back:

- *The Posterior Longitudinal Ligament (PLL)*—a long strip down running all the way down the *front part* of the spinal canal. This ligament drapes down from your head to your tailbone, connects to the discs, and looks a little bit like a kite-tail.

- *The Ligamentum Flavum*—not one long ligament, but many delightfully moth-shaped ligaments connecting each spine bone to another. These shiny, yellowish little fancies inhabit the *back part* of the spinal canal. When you stand up straight or bend backward, the healthy *ligamentum flavum's* elasticity keeps it from buckling into the *spinal canal.*

Think of the ligaments in your own spine. Are they in good condition, pressed, hanging neatly in place? Or are they frayed, wadded, or bunched in a pile? Has your ligamentum flavum lost a bit of elasticity? Does it buckle in toward your spinal canal when you try to stand up straight? The answer is most likely related to your overall physical health. Do you get some type of regular aerobic exercise? Do you have diabetes? Do you smoke? Do you eat a healthy diet? And so on.

Once ligaments are damaged, can their health improve? Yes. The health of your ligaments is something you may have control over.

Changes in Connective Tissue (fascia)

A beautiful substance, with the ability to both expand and contract, fascia is this moist, elastic cobwebby stuff that permeates our bodies and basically connects... well, just everything. There are many different types of fascia throughout the human body and their consistencies (sometimes feathery, sometimes dense) and functions change depending on where they are located. The fascia between muscles helps them glide as they contract. With prolonged stress, lack of movement, poor circulation, and altered metabolism, various fasciae can become rigid, tight, restrictive, or inflamed.

Is it possible to change the health of your own fascia? Of course, it is! Stretching, relaxing, and deep breathing exercises are a great place to start.

Swelling

Blobs of fluid accumulate in and around your tissues in response to inflammation. Swelling can take up space in your spinal canal, leaving less room for your spinal cord and nerves.

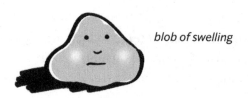

blob of swelling

Of all the things hogging space in your spinal canal, swelling is perhaps the easiest to reduce. Hence, I like to think of swelling as the spinal stenosis "X factor." How important is it for someone with stenosis to decrease inflammation? So important it's the first "Focus Area" you'll read about in Part Two.

Take your Anatomy (and your MRI results) with a Grain of Salt

Anatomical diagrams can be helpful, but they can also be misleading. If your MRI shows a severe disc protrusion or a spur, you may believe (based on your knowledge of anatomy) this spur or disc is pushing on your spinal cord, and that you will never get rid of your pain unless a surgeon removes it. But 80% of people with MRIs showing spurs or disc bulges have few or no symptoms at all.

Yes, you may have a disc protrusion. Yes, you may have a pretty big spur or two. You may even have one vertebra sitting right on top of the other in a "bone-on-bone" type of situation, or one bone slipped forward or fusing itself into the other. None of these conditions guarantees you'll have pain, numbness, or weakness.

How is this possible? Well, it might not be *that* bone spur or *that* disc bulge pushing on the nerve. It might be a big blob of swelling around that spur or disc bulge. It might be that your overall circulation is so bad the nerve isn't getting an adequate blood supply. It might be that an enlarged ligament takes up so much space it pushes your spinal cord into that spur or disc bulge.

> One day, an 85-year-old woman came hobbling into my clinic. I took one look at "Helen" and wondered, How can I possibly help this person? She had very severe scoliosis (a condition in which the top half of the spine curves to one side, and the bottom part curves to the other) and severe degenerative joint disease. Her spine was hunched and twisted like a corkscrew.
>
> "What part of you hurts the most?" I asked.
>
> "Oh, I don't have any pain at all—it's just my balance that's off."
>
> "Are you kidding me?" I said.
>
> This woman had collapsed vertebrae, bony deformities, spurs, and disc protrusions all over the place. But she had exactly Z-E-R-O pain. How did she do it?

I don't have a definitive answer to that, but I can tell you what I observed. Helen seemed to be in almost constant motion. She was an animated speaker, shifting forward or back in her chair, and turning this way or that to make a point. This constant movement must've been great for her overall circulation. She was also very optimistic about her ability to make improvements. Thirdly, despite her age, she had no real health problems—no diabetes, no high blood pressure, no obesity. She was a non-smoker, got lots of exercise, and slept like a baby.

Positive attitude, exercise, good overall wellness-level, and a habit for activity over couch potato-ism. Sounds like a pretty good formula for success.

Many of the problems of spinal stenosis (and, hence, most of the solutions) have to do with what's happening on a cellular level. By this, I mean the quality of your circulation, cell metabolism, and overall tissue health.

Am I saying anatomy isn't important? No.

Am I saying your MRI results aren't important? No.

I am saying that neither is the be-all and end-all.

As Seattle spine surgeon Alexis Falikov reminded me: "We don't treat x-rays and we don't treat MRI's. We treat symptoms."

It may help to think of your spinal canal as a big, cluttered-up laundry chute with a very delicate conductive cable running right through the center of it. Your job, in rehabilitating yourself, is to de-clutter this laundry chute without needing to have a surgeon do it.

HOW SPINAL STENOSIS DIFFERS FROM ORDINARY LOW BACK PAIN

When it comes to treatment for back pain, people are full of advice—but spinal stenosis is different from run-of-the-mill back pain. First of all, walking is considered the crème-de-la-crème of back exercises. But walking long distances often makes spinal stenosis symptoms worse, putting more pressure on the spinal cord or nerve roots and causing weakening rather than strengthening of the legs and back muscles. I won't say it's impossible or even completely unadvisable to use walking as your primary exercise when you have spinal stenosis, but in many cases it is not the best first choice.

Ordinary back pain does not give you neurogenic claudication—a fancy name for that annoying weakness, numbness, and cramping in your legs.

Ordinary back pain does not generally feel better when you sit down. With spinal stenosis, sitting down often provides immediate relief.

Ordinary back pain most often feels worse with bending. Stenotics can often touch their toes with ease. In fact, bending forward often makes it feel better.

Ordinary Low Back Pain vs. Spinal Stenosis

Ordinary Low Back Pain	Spinal Stenosis
Worse with bending forward.	Often not worse with bending forward.
No relief with sitting.	Sitting provides fast relief.
Pain with sneezing or coughing.	No pain with sneezing or coughing.
No unnatural heaviness or buckling in legs.	Unnatural heavy-legs feeling in standing.
Often eased by standing up straighter.	Often feels worse when standing up straighter.
Strength in legs does not vary with position.	Less leg weakness when sitting or lying down.

It's important to keep in mind that some common exercises for ordinary low back pain can aggravate spinal stenosis. Certain movements, especially end-range twisting or bending backward, can decrease space in the spinal canal and nerve openings, causing structures to clamp down on nerves or the spinal cord. While not everyone will be aggravated (or helped) by the same exercises, it pays to know what to be careful of when figuring out your exercise plan.

SUMMARY

- Spinal stenosis is caused by many different factors—not just bone or discs.
- Many aspects of spinal stenosis can be changed:

    - Swelling and inflammation in and around the spine
    - Health of joints, fascia, discs, and ligaments of the spine
    - Circulation (or blood supply) to the spine
    - Functional strength of muscles supporting the spine

- How you feel is more important than how bad the X-ray or MRI looks. You can have severe stenosis with mild symptoms, and you can have mild stenosis with severe symptoms.
- Some things that are helpful for ordinary low back pain (including some exercises) are not very helpful for spinal stenosis.

SAFETY TIPS

DON'T try to diagnose your own spinal stenosis. A physician should help you determine the cause of your particular symptoms.

DON'T force yourself to stand up straight if it makes your legs feel weaker.

DO see a doctor immediately if you have any of the following red flags:

- Loss of bowel or bladder control or numbness in the genital region.
- Sudden severe, unrelenting low back pain.
- Any unusual weight loss or weight gain.
- Foot is dragging on the floor when you walk ("drop foot").
- Any rapidly progressing weakness, numbness, or tingling.

FAKE, BUT USEFUL... SPINAL STENOSIS TERMS

Spinal Stenocrust: **crusty spurs around the edge of your spine bones.**
"Hey, Joe. Your X-rays showed a few small spurs here and there in the low lumbar region. Nothing to worry about, just a little spinal stenocrust."

Spinal Stenostressed: **all stressed out about spinal stenosis.**
"You want me to stand up straight? I'm so spinal stenostressed, I can't even think straight!"

Spinal Stenoplus: **anything good for spinal stenosis.**
"Increasing circulation is a big spinal stenoplus."

PART TWO

Three Focus Areas

Each of the next three sections highlights a different focus area. **Focus Area 1** teaches you how to control inflammation and swelling. **Focus Area 2** introduces exercises specifically helpful for spinal stenosis. **Focus Area 3** reveals the wellness changes crucial to restoring the health of your spine.

Though these focus areas are numbered, they are not to be applied in any particular order, nor are they mutually exclusive. Following the instructions in one focus area will only enhance results from the instructions in another focus area. In planning your rehab program, the best approach is to gather tips from each category into a sort of "stenosis toolbox." Pull out one or two when you need them. Others can be part of your daily routine.

Decrease Inflammation

< FOCUS AREA 1 >

JILL JOHNSON'S ANKLE

When amateur triathlete, Jill "Willpower" Johnson, sprains her ankle on a jagged sidewalk, what happens? Her ankle becomes inflamed and swollen. The swelling takes up space in the ankle, and if Jill never ices it or takes care of it, the inflammation becomes *chronic.* (In other words, it lasts way longer than it needs to.) Jill's ankle gets thick and shiny and, if you poke a finger into it, a thimble-sized divot appears and stays for several seconds. When you traumatize your spine, the same type of swelling happens. This swelling, however, lives deep in the joints.

You can't usually see it, but you can almost always feel it.

WHAT IT'S LIKE TO HAVE SWELLING

Imagine somebody just cracked open a couple of eggs and let the contents seep into the base of your spine. At first, the egg-stuff is runny and liquidy, but the longer it sits there, the thicker and globbier it gets. What we're basically dealing with here is a bunch of extra fluid and white blood cells taking up space between the joints of your spine. Like a bad tenant, the longer your swelling stays, the harder it is to get rid of. The extra fluid takes up room, room that could be used for good tenants, like nerves, blood vessels, ligaments etc... But wait, it gets worse. Swelling doesn't just take up space, it *infiltrates* the "good tenants" (ligaments, muscles, fascia, etc...), thickens them and hardens them, and depletes their elasticity. And if that isn't bad enough, inflammation releases tiny chemical irritants that actually make you hurt! Imagine wicked little gremlins, splashing buckets of hydrochloric acid around— this is how inflammation totally messes with your tissues.

Of course, there are no gremlins and this excess fluid doesn't come from cracked eggs.

It comes from inside your own body.

It's easy to think of stenosis as coming from some bone or disc pushing directly on a nerve or the spinal cord, but these structures can often just bend around that bone or disc, as long as there's enough space.

What reduces space? Swelling.

Can you shrink a bone yourself? Pretty tough—not sure it's possible.

Can you shrink a disc protrusion? Sometimes.

Can you shrink the inflammation of all the structures of your spine? Of course!

COMMON SIGNS OF INFLAMMATION

What if I don't have any inflammation in my spine? How can I tell if it's there or not? Common signs of low back inflammation include:

- a feeling of heat over the spine
- constant severe pain or aching
- sleep disturbed by pain
- pain with standing or walking more than a few minutes
- pain with turning in bed or changing position
- pain getting up from a chair
- pain with any quick movements
- the sudden worsening of symptoms (known as a "flare-up")

**ALWAYS CONSULT YOUR PHYSICIAN WITH ANY
SUDDEN WORSENING OF LOW BACK PAIN.**

Rather than trying to figure out whether inflammation is adding to your symptoms, you could follow the instructions in this chapter and see if there's a change. Give it a good five days. You may be surprised by how much it helps.

TAKE GOOD CARE OF YOUR INFLAMED SPINE

Let's go back to Jill Johnson and her sprained swollen ankle. If she wanted to take good care of herself, how would she go about it? She might elevate her ankle, ice it several times a day, and wrap it with an ACE bandage. If it's a bad sprain, she'll use crutches for a bit till she feels like she can bear more weight. She'd certainly want to avoid aggravating activities like sprinting, jumping, making sharp cuts, or skiing for a while. But should she stop moving it entirely? Actually, Jill will be better off doing some gentle movements and light strengthening—nothing too vigorous—just enough to keep it moving. Once she's feeling better, she can gradually reintroduce things like walking, skipping, and jogging.

In the same way, you can use these "Eight Anti-Inflammatory Strategies" to take good care of your inflamed spine.

1. Find Your Best Resting Positions
2. Use Ice
3. Protect Your Spine with a Lumbar Corset
4. Unload your Spine with Assistive Walking Devices
5. Avoid Aggravating Positions, Activities, and Heavy Lifting
6. Gradually Re-introduce Activities as You Start to Feel Better
7. Use Good Body Mechanics
8. Keep Exercising (even if it's just a little!)

ANTI-INFLAMMATORY STRATEGY #1:
Find Your Best Resting Positions

Finding (and using!) the best resting positions for your spine is the closest analogy I can think of to elevating a sprained ankle. Imagine your spine, perfectly aligned, in an unloaded position: No kinked joints, minimized pressure, and very little pain. You're able to breathe more deeply, stimulating your lymphatic system to reduce local swelling. For anyone in constant pain, I recommend finding and getting into your best rest position for 15 to 30 minutes, two to four times per day.

What are the best resting positions for lumbar spinal stenosis? The first rule is to pay attention to whatever most relieves your symptoms. Certain positions, however, tend to be more comfortable and take a load off the spine. They are:

- Side-lying with a pillow between the knees and another pillow hugged to the chest.

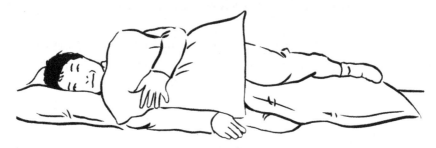

- Lying on your back with pillows under the upper back (or some kind of wedge under the shoulders) with pillows (or an ottoman) under the knees.

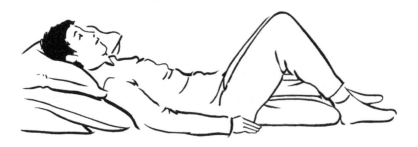

- Reclining in a recliner.
- Soaking in a pool or hot tub.
- Just sitting down for a few minutes.

What's so great about these positions? Well, there seems to be more room for the spinal cord when the spine is bent (flexed). This is why you see people with spinal stenosis walking bent over—they're trying to create space for the spinal cord so the nerves keep firing to their legs. Because of this, lying flat on your back or on your stomach can be really uncomfortable.

When lying on your side, use pillows

- in front of you,
- behind you, and
- between your knees.

This helps prevent subtle but painful twists and rotations.

Of course, the body needs movement to maintain adequate circulation, strength, and mobility, so spending too much time in one position is not a good idea. Positioning yourself to reduce inflammation should be done in moderation. Getting into a position of comfort and staying in it all day? Probably *not* a good idea. Getting into a position of comfort for fifteen minutes to a half-hour, three to four times per day? Now *this* is an excellent idea.

ANTI-INFLAMMATORY STRATEGY #2:
Use Ice

Funny how the strategy people are most reluctant to try is also the strategy that can give the most relief. Many of my clients have trouble with the idea of putting a freezing cold anything anywhere, let alone on their low back. I can't even count the number of times I've heard the line, "I hate ice—it's so...cold."

But if you can just get over the initial shock of it, I'm telling you, ice works wonders for spinal stenosis.

Ice is Nice

There are three ways ice helps pain from spinal stenosis:

1. Increases circulation to the deepest parts of your back.
2. Slows the conduction of pain signals to the brain (woo hoo!).
3. Reduces the heat associated with inflammation.

During periods of flare-up, I recommend using 10 minutes of ice *at least* twice daily, and up to four times daily, for one week. By the end of the week, you and your stenosis will be in a better place.

How Ice Works

Using ice for just ten minutes improves blood flow to your spine. You've heard of hypothermia. A person exposed to extreme cold in the wilderness goes into shock. In this state, the superficial blood vessels constrict and the deeper blood vessels open up, shunting blood to the vital organs needed for survival.

When you apply ice to your low back, you essentially trick your body into a sort of localized hypothermia. Deep spinal muscles and joints receive a nice, much-needed infusion of blood and nutrients. The result is a reduction in spasm and a groovy deep muscle relaxation. This is only the first of the awesome things ice does for you.

Using ice for just ten minutes reduces the level of your pain. Lower temperatures slow things down—and this includes nerve conduction. Basically, it's too darn cold for the nerve to send those angry pain signals up the spinal cord to the brain.

Aren't you going to fire your pain signal?

No, it's too darn cold!

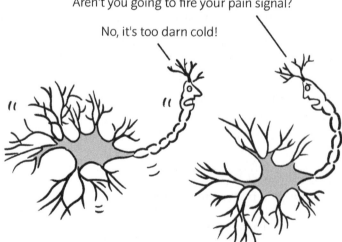

Pain signals travel along the spinal cord to the brain. When a nerve cell fires a pain signal, it travels at a certain rate:

SOS SOS SOS SOS SOS.

If the pain is more intense, the signal travels along a little faster:

SOS SOS SOS SOS.

Pain is like a pot of simmering water. If you add heat to your aching back, the water simmers faster or starts boiling.

SOSOSOSOSOSOSOSSSSSSSS!!!!!!

Take the heat away and it calms down. Put ICE in the water and the boiling slows to a stop.

SOS...S....O.....

If you are in constant, severe low back pain, using ice can give you relief.

Using ice for just ten minutes reduces the heat of inflammation. Why would NBA Champion and Cleveland Cavaliers star LeBron James dunk his hot, swollen ankles in a big tub of ice water after a big game? To cool them down, of course.

And reduce the *heat* of inflammation.

How to Use Ice Correctly

- *Use ice without a lot of layers in between.* A single pillowcase or paper towel is enough to protect your skin. A towel is probably too much layering and will not provide the full effect. Your ice pack should be *cold,* not just *cool.*

- *An ice pack should be left on no more than 10 minutes.* This prevents frostbite. Use a timer with an alarm to prevent yourself from forgetting or falling asleep.

- *Use soft ice*—a soft ice pack conforms to your body's contours. (That old-fashioned clunky ice bag can help a little, but sometimes you want your cold therapy to cover more than just a few inches.) I recommend buying a gel pack from the local pharmacy or you can order a couple on-line.

- *Use strategic ice.* Always ice over the center of your spine, but it may help to try it out on other areas too (right butt cheek, outside of the thigh, etc...). Always use ice in a position of comfort.

- *Never use ice over an area of numbness.* This precaution also helps to prevent frostbite.

Always Use Ice in a Position of Comfort

- Lie on it with your feet up on a chair, bolster, or sofa (a.k.a. the 90/90 position) or just with a few pillows under your knees.
- Lie on your side with a pillow between your knees and strap it to yourself using a sheet, elastic-waist pants, or a lumbar corset (see next section) Get your grandkid to hold it on!
- Lie on it in your groovy faux-leather recliner!

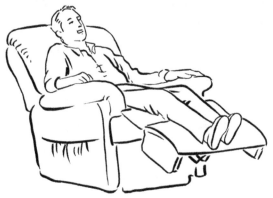

USE YOUR ICE PACK FOR 10 MINUTES

Different Types of Ice Packs

- *Gel packs.* Best for conforming to your body's contours. Buy in a medical supply store, local pharmacy, or on-line.
- *Frozen vegetables* (peas, corn, or black-eyed peas). Inexpensive option, but can be lumpy and uncomfortable. May work better if you spread them out inside a one-gallon Ziploc bag.
- *Homemade "slushy" pack.* Use two-parts water mixed with one part rubbing alcohol inside two Ziploc bags (do not overfill) or a hot water bottle. *Warning: the homemade slushy pack is colder than normal ice, so you need to add an extra layer to prevent frostbite.

Try an Ice Massage

(Almost as good as a nice massage!)

Truly my favorite type of coldness—it's fast, it's effective...what's not to love? Take some small paper cups, fill them with water, and freeze. Peel back the top of one of the cups, exposing about a quarter-inch of the ice. Then get someone nice to massage it around your spine, buttock, or even part of your leg. For comfort's sake, stick to one 3-4 inch square area at a time. (Don't be too surprised if it feels unbelievably cold at first. You'll adjust to it fairly quickly and the payoff is huge!) Use strategically placed towels to catch renegade drips. If your helper is really nice, he or she can dab you dry with a cloth after every 4-5 swipes of this delectable frozen therapy. *To avoid frostbite, keep treatment limited to 3-5 minutes.*

The Ideal Icy Reception

Hate the idea of putting ice on your spine? Imagine your back is on fire, or maybe a burning boiling cauldron. As the ice comes into contact with your skin, imagine the sound of a hot skillet being plunged into cold water. Ssssss. Ahhhhh.

ANTI-INFLAMMATORY STRATEGY #3:
Protect Your Spine with a Lumbar Corset

Let's get back to Jill Johnson and her big, fat sprained ankle. Jill's doctor has advised her to wrap it with an ACE bandage. The bandage compresses out the swelling, and keeps the ankle supported to prevent re-injury.

Take this analogy and apply it to your spine. Your ACE bandage equivalent is the elastic lumbar corset:

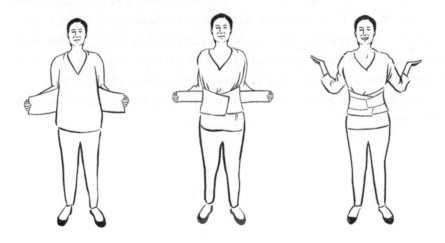

What does a lumbar corset do?

- Reduces strain and repetitive large side-bending movements
- Unloads the spine by as much as 20%
- Allows you to stay active while preventing further injury

A corset is more or less a passive technique. Once you put it on, you don't really have to think about it and it more or less does its job.

When it comes to lumbar corsets, I prefer the elastic ones. Elastic corsets are not rigid. They don't prevent *ALL* movements like a body cast or lace-up corset. They prevent *DRAMATIC* movements. How? Just by sending your body a little feedback. Everybody benefits from a little feedback, right?

Many people are shy of corsets and back braces...

Won't that just make me weak?

Well, yes—and no. It *will* make you weak if you wear it *all the time* (you'll become dependent on it and stop using your muscles properly). It *won't* make you weak, if you wear it *off and on* (maybe when you're in the kitchen, or doing some other activity, or just for 30 minutes at a time 3x per day) or if you use it to *sleep* in.

How Can a Corset Help Me While I Sleep?

Humans normally change position between 3 to 72 times per night. If you have pain when you turn in bed, or if you wake up sore in the morning, wearing a corset to sleep may help. It works by stabilizing your low back, and encouraging you to use other parts of your body to twist (such as your upper back and hips). In this way, a corset can actually make you more flexible. And when you no longer have to guard against painful movements, your relaxation level, breathing, and circulation improve. What's not to like about a better night's sleep?

Now, are you sure a corset won't make me weak?

Perfectly sure. When used right, a corset actually helps you to become strong. Again, your first goal is to reduce pain and inflammation. It's OK to use a corset whenever your symptoms are severe. (When you're feeling better, you can stick it in your dresser drawer and forget about it.) And it's OK to use a corset when you're taking a long walk. If you can walk 15 minutes before having to sit down *without a corset* and 30 minutes *with a corset*, which practice do you think provides a better cardio workout?

ANTI-INFLAMMATORY STRATEGY #4:
Unload Your Spine with Assistive Walking Devices

Let's get back to our intrepid ankle sprain sufferer...

Jill ACE-wrapped her ankle, but it still hurts to walk on it. What else can she do to protect that joint while the swelling goes down? She can use *crutches*. Crutches help Jill keep the weight off the ankle. She can hop around on them, keeping her foot hanging in the air, or just use them to keep a little weight off the ankle while she walks.

Just as Jill uses crutches to keep the weight off her injured ankle, you can use some kind of device, be it a cane, walker, or trekking poles, to keep some pressure off your spine. Much like the corset, assistive walking devices are tools, and tools are used on an as-needed basis. The goal is to make you more independent and keep yourself moving.

Time to Dust off the old W-A-L-K-E-R

The mere word inspires an expression at once fearful and hostile. The eyes widen. The body becomes tense. It is a look that begs: *Don't say that.... Please, don't say that....*

WALKER! WALKER! WALKER! OK, I said it.

The front-wheeled walker (a walker with wheels in front, often with tennis balls plunked onto the back legs) is a symbol of one's last long traversal to the, ahem, ultimate resting place. Nothing says "face-it, you're old" like pushing an assemblage of aluminum piping on wheels. Right?

Wrong.

If you have spinal stenosis, and your legs have given out on you, then you should own a walker.

If you have spinal stenosis, and you have fallen due to leg weakness, you should have a walker.

Many people refuse to use them. If this is you, and you are just being stubborn about your very serious loss of strength in the legs, you can walk even shorter distances and are more likely to fall, break a hip, and wind up in a nursing home than your less prideful/paranoid counterparts.

Does owning a walker mean your life is over? No. Does it mean you always have to use it? No. Many people with stenosis find that if they use a walker for longer excursions, or exclusively for 2-3 days at a time when their symptoms flare-up, they can ditch the walker later. Some use a walker only in the morning when they're stiff, some at the end of the day when they're tired.

NUMBER ONE REASON TO OWN A WALKER:
WALKERS PREVENT FALLS

Falls are bad. Falls can lead to hip fractures, but they can also lead to *compression fractures* in the spine. A compression fracture alters your spine bone from its normal cube-shape into a wedge- or triangle-shape (see page 26). They are quite painful and the wedge-shaped bone makes you stoop even more. Even if you don't break something, a fall can lead to increased inflammation, humiliation, and a traumatic event for the whole family. If your legs are buckling on you, chances are a walker can prevent you from falling.

Whether you think you're ready for a walker or not, the reality is, in cases of severe pain or weakness, a walker works to keep you moving. It works to keep the load off your spine, which reduces the inflammation and encourages the health of discs. Let me say again: Walkers prevent falls. Falls make stenosis worse. Falls can lead to broken bones.

NUMBER TWO REASON TO OWN A WALKER:
WALKERS ALLOW YOU TO KEEP MOVING

Walkers normalize gait, so you don't have to limp. Limping puts lopsided pressures on the spine and joints. Limping increases joint inflammation and pressure on the nerves.

Movement is essential for circulation. Circulation is essential for healing and reduction of inflammation. Movement is essential for full body health.

Years ago, I used a walker for a bit after I injured my back doing martial arts. Was it a little embarrassing? Sure. (OK, fine, it was *a lot* embarrassing.) But I could barely stand, and that thing got me moving again. I was off it in five days, and without it my rehab would have taken much longer.

ANTI-INFLAMMATORY STRATEGY #5:
Avoid Aggravating Positions, Activities, and Heavy Lifting

Just as it is important to know your best rest positions, you should also know the positions and movements that aggravate your stenosis—and avoid them during periods of inflammatory flare-up.

Aggravating Positions for Spinal Stenosis

- Lying on your stomach (may feel better with a pillow under your tummy and feet)
- Lying flat on your back (may feel better with a pillow under your knees)
- Prolonged standing or being on your feet
- Forcing yourself to stand up straight when you feel more comfortable stooping

Aggravating Activities for Spinal Stenosis

- *Extension (bending backwards)* Bending backwards narrows the nerve exit-holes in your spine, and creates less room for the spinal cord. Examples of spinal extension include:
  - Reaching up to change a light-bulb
  - Drinking a glass of water while standing (ouch!)
  - Lying on your stomach, propped on your elbows
  - Washing windows (reaching up is a killer!)
  - Casting a fishing line
  - Walking downstairs or downhill
  - Standing or walking in a more erect position than is normal for you

- *Twisting* Twisting repeatedly, *especially through large movements*, can create friction, irritation, and increased swelling. Examples of repetitive twisting include:
  - Loading the dishwasher
  - Vacuuming
  - Dropping your knees from side to side to "stretch out" your back
  - Elliptical trainer
  - Weeding

- Pruning rose bushes
- Tennis
- Casting a fishing line
- Washing windows
- Throwing a ball
- Unpacking boxes

While a person with stenosis may be able to comfortably perform some or all of these activities, you'll want to avoid them until your symptoms are better.

Heavy Lifting

Can a person with lumbar spinal stenosis ever do heavy lifting? Many can and do this without much problem at all. *However,* when your back is hurting, or you are flared up and having trouble standing in the kitchen to cook a meal, I don't recommend helping a friend move his refrigerator down a flight of stairs, digging an irrigation ditch in the backyard, or even carrying around your already-walking-fine-on-his-own two-year-old grandson.

Don't Let Yourself Get Pushed Around
—or Upright—by Well-Meaning Friends

If you're walking and someone tries to force you into a more upright position, resist your first impulse to do something violent. This uninformed person is only trying to help. Try this:

"Thank you for trying to help me. You know, I think what I really need is to sit down for a moment."

Or maybe:

"I know you mean well, but it's actually bad to force someone with spinal stenosis into an upright position. What you're doing is going to injure me."

Of course, it's possible you could be standing more bent over than you need to. So your best bet might be to periodically check in with your body to see if standing upright really does increase the weakness in your legs. If it doesn't make your legs weak, why not go for it?

Keep a Checklist

It'd be nice if everyone with spinal stenosis had the same symptoms, aggravated by exactly the same activities. Then I could give you a blanket list of do's and don'ts and we wouldn't have to worry about anything else. Unfortunately (or fortunately depending on your perspective) everybody's just a little bit different, which is why the above-listed activities are only guidelines, *likely* to flare you up, not *guaranteed* to flare you up. I recommend avoiding these activities when your symptoms are severe, trying them a little bit at a time when your symptoms are less severe—and if they flare you up every time (give it 24-48 hours before you decide), cross them off your list. For now, at least.

Posting your own list of aggravating activities on the refrigerator or bathroom mirror is a great way to reinforce good inflammation control.

ANTI-INFLAMMATORY STRATEGY #6:
Gradually Reintroduce Activities as You Start to Feel Better

Once you've put some time and effort into reducing inflammation, you should begin to see some improvements. Some of these include:

- Feeling more comfortable getting in and out of bed
- Decreased burning or heat in your back or legs
- Pain is no longer severe or constant
- Sleep is not disturbed by pain (turning in bed feels fine)
- Feeling more comfortable standing or walking
- No pain getting up from a chair
- No pain with any quick movements (you no longer feel like you have to guard)
- You're standing up a little straighter—and it's just coming naturally to you

When you have achieved these things, you can begin to reintroduce some of the activities you've put on hold. Wait! Don't make the mistake of jumping right back in to *everything* you were doing before! Pick one or two things to try and see how it goes. And you'll probably need to change the way you do them, too—using less aggravating techniques so you don't flare yourself up. The techniques and strategies used to protect your spine during activities fall under the category of "good body mechanics."

ANTI-INFLAMMATORY STRATEGY #7:
Use Good Body Mechanics

Efficient movement is truly an art. In sports it's called "good form." But to us non-jocks, trying to get something accomplished in the kitchen, garage, or garden, it's called "good body mechanics." Teaching people to use good body mechanics has been a staple of physical therapists for years. Almost everyone who has ever worked for a large company went through body mechanics instruction as part of their "New Hire Orientation Program," and it always hammers home the same simple points:

- Don't *bend at the waist*—bend at the knees.
- Lift with your legs.
- Pivot, don't twist.
- Push, don't pull.

These are good tips, but they are also incomplete. Back in the early '90s, I taught an Introductory Back Class for Kaiser Permanente in San Francisco. Patients who had back pain were "invited" to attend two 90-minute sessions before they could even see a physical therapist one-on-one. This made for a very grumpy group of San Franciscans on the first day of back class. Slouched in their hard plastic stackable chairs, arms folded across their chests, my poor trapped audience waited for the inevitable boring lecture. Almost each and every face said the same thing: *This is going to be a big waste of time. I've already heard all this stuff.*

And I just have to tell you, I've come to love this type of audience.

After going over a little bit of spine anatomy (all while fantasizing lightly of being off somewhere else having a pack of Hostess chocolate Donettes), I'd suddenly drop to the floor...a copy of the huge and heavy *Grey's Atlas of Human Anatomy*. Whump!

"OK, folks, let's say I'm going to have to lift this book for work. Tell me how I should do it."

"Bend your knees!" someone would shout.

"Don't bend at the waist!" would cry another.

"Well," I'd say. "Is that all you've got?"

"Brace your stomach muscles?"

Then silence.

"That's *it*?"

More silence.

"OK," I'd say. "How about my feet?"

"Apart!"

"How far apart?"

The whole class in unison: "Shoulder-width!"

"Shoulder-width?"

"Yes!!"

The Joy of a Super Wide Stance

Perhaps you, the reader, are savvy. Perhaps you know the right answer isn't *shoulder-width* apart. No, the feet must be *wider than shoulder-width* apart. Because without your feet being wider than shoulder-width apart, bending your knees isn't going to help much.

Try this:

1. Place something light—maybe a pen—on the floor in front of you. Stand in front of the pen with your feet *shoulder-width* apart. Now, bend your knees and pick up the pen.

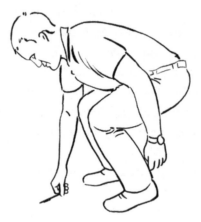

2. Next try the same thing with your feet *wider than shoulder-width* apart. The first thing you'll notice is, the more your feet go apart, the lower you are and the *closer* you are to the pen. The second thing you'll notice is, you don't have to reach *over your knees* to get to the silly thing. You can basically straddle it, right?

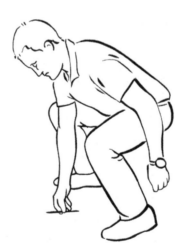

See how the wider than shoulder-width stance gets your knees out of the way? See how it lets you bend at the hips more easily? See how the guy in the second picture looks more balanced? Well, he doesn't just *look* more balanced. He *is* more balanced.

If the wider than shoulder-width stance were only good for lifting things, maybe I wouldn't be quite so in love with it. But this trick is good for lots of things! It even comes in handy with hateful chores like the dishes.

Here's an experiment to try in the kitchen:

1. Bend and touch the bottom of the sink with your feet merely shoulder-width apart.

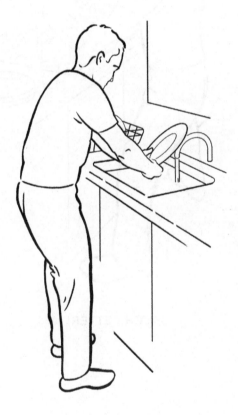

AHEM. NOT GOOD.

2. Then bend and touch the bottom of the sink with your feet *wider than shoulder-width.* Which feels better? Multiply your "better feeling" by the number of times you reach into the sink while doing dishes.

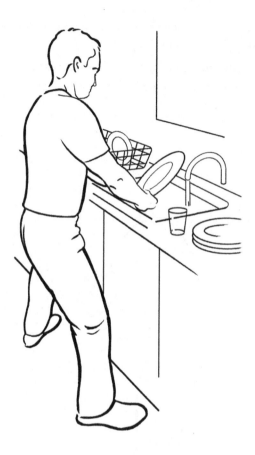

MUCH BETTER!

3. Now reach into the sink with your knees shoulder-width and place an imaginary dish into the dish drainer (or dish washer).

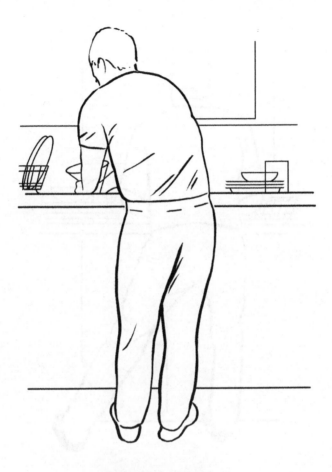

UGH. NOT GOOD.

4. Then switch to your super-wide stance. As you put the dish into the drainer, shift your weight onto the leg closest to the dish drainer and bend the knee slightly. What's different? How much twisting did your spine have to do with each method?

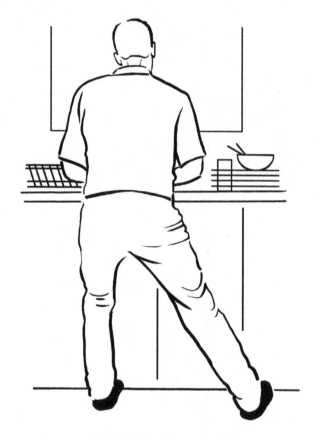

THIS IS SUPER GOOD!

Your feet are your first (and mostly your only) contact with the ground. Everything you do with your body depends heavily on the position of your feet. A super-wide stance lets you use your whole body, not just your spine.

The Golfer's Tee Trick

This nifty technique requires a bit of practice, and a fairly decent sense of balance, but is definitely worth learning for the safe retrieval of some light object off the floor, such as the just-dropped pen, odd bit of change, or piece of candy. The trick basically consists of turning yourself into a human teeter-totter by kicking one leg up behind you, while you reach toward the floor. Once you have what you want, the weight of your leg helps bring you back up.

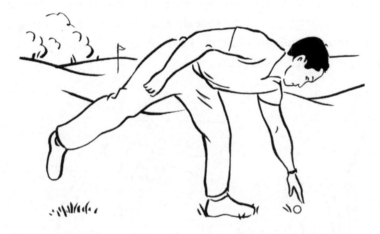

The beauty of this maneuver is that it can be incorporated into any sort of reaching, for any sort of light object, at any height. Need to snatch something yummy from the back of the kitchen counter? Piece of cake! Need to grab a screwdriver from the far end of your workbench? You now have the perfect tool! Want to plug something in? It's electrifyingly easy!

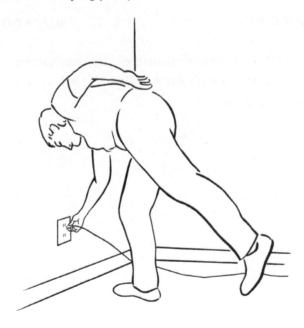

The Lunge

The "lunge" is really a very close relative of the "golfer's tee trick." Being able to do a good lunge is a great way to protect your spine.

Unlike the golfer's tee trick and the super-wide stance, the lunge can be a bit more stressful on the knees. However, everyone can use the movement of a lunge to make everyday activities easier on the spine.

For example, many people have more pain and symptoms when they're standing at the sink to shave or put on make-up, leaning close to the mirror so they can see what they're doing. Just spitting in the sink after some nice tooth-brushing can be problematic. My recommendation for these kinds of activities: When you do a little bend, *always put one leg behind you.*

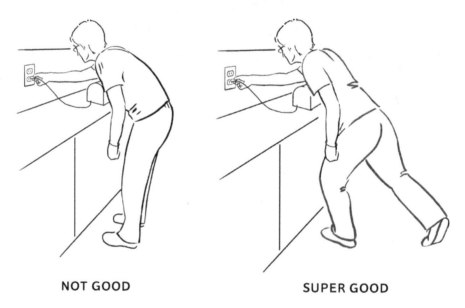

NOT GOOD   **SUPER GOOD**

Oh, yeah, and if you have more pain in one leg than another, when doing a lunge or golfer's tee trick, *always put the painful leg in back.* This shifts the weight to the stronger or less painful side.

Getting Out of Bed

Vaulting up out of bed might be invigorating, but when the low back is inflamed, it can also be painful and aggravating. To reduce strain on the back, draw one knee up at a time and curl up into a comfy ball as you roll on to your side. Drop your legs over the edge of the bed and push yourself into a sitting position.

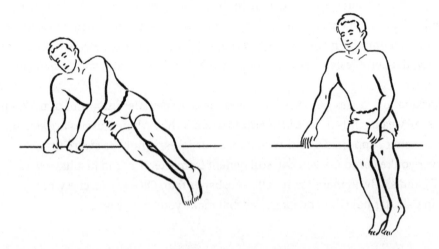

DON'T BE A ROBOT

Some of us believe that the best way to protect the spine is to move like a robot. We walk around like a robot. Lift things like a robot (knees shoulder-width apart). Make love like a robot and so on. But the fact is, human beings are not robots. It's normal for us to move in multiple directions: multiple planes, diagonals, and spirals. We need rotation in our spines when we walk to promote healthy circulation and normal tissue elasticity.

If your focus is on treating inflammation, you should avoid *extreme* rotational or repetitive *large* rotational movements—but don't tense up and stop moving like a normal person—let those arms and shoulders swing when you walk! Breathe deeply and try to relax.

ANTI-INFLAMMATORY STRATEGY #8:
Keep Exercising (even if it's just a little!)

It may be shocking to discover the notion of *exercise* in a chapter on reducing inflammation. *How can I exercise if my spine is inflamed? Isn't that dangerous?*

Actually, it's dangerous to completely *stop* exercising.

Did you know exercise actually reduces inflammation? It's true! During exercise, anti-inflammatory molecules circulate through your tissues—while molecules promoting inflammation are reduced. Perhaps this is why people who get some type of regular aerobic exercise are much less likely to suffer from spinal stenosis symptoms.

Inflammation causes weakness, and weakness perpetuates inflammation. When muscles are weak, joints don't line up quite so smoothly. When muscles are strong, joints are better supported. For this chapter's purposes, simply be aware that, whenever you're flared up, you can still benefit from exercise. You just have to do it carefully and safely. Remember, it's OK—no, better than OK—to exercise when you're in pain; it's not OK to do exercises that make your pain worse.

> REMEMBER, IT'S OK TO EXERCISE WHEN YOU'RE IN PAIN;
> IT'S NOT OK TO DO EXERCISES THAT MAKE YOUR PAIN WORSE.

How to Safely Exercise

When your symptoms are flared up, it's safest to exercise only in those positions of maximum comfort. These can be some of the positions I've listed earlier or some you've discovered on your own. (Remember, there are no "wrong" positions as long as they're comfortable to you.) Stick to beginner level exercises—incorporating fewer reps and lower amounts of resistance—to move past an inflammatory cycle.

The next focus area describes some of my favorite spinal stenosis exercises. Many are presented from beginner-level, to intermediate-level, to advanced-level. All beginner-level exercises are described in one of the best rest positions or "easing" positions for spinal stenosis. When your symptoms are severe, and to keep inflammation to a minimum, start with only the beginner-level exercises and progress from there. Rule of Thumb: if you try a new exercise and it doesn't make you worse over the next few days, it's probably OK to keep on doing it.

As you consider beginning some of the exercises in the next chapter, keep in mind that no exercise has to be done at 100% effort. You can start by contracting your muscles at 50% or even 25% effort. If there's no flare-up after a few days, you can put more into it.

Just Five Days...

Motivating yourself to control inflammation can be tough. Maybe it's because doing protective things makes you feel disabled. Maybe you don't like (or aren't used to) pampering yourself. Whatever the reasons, I've witnessed a lot of resistance from people in my years as a therapist:

- "I don't have time to rest; I've got too many things to do."
- "I don't want to use a walker—it makes me feel old, and besides, once I get on it, I'll never get off."
- "Ice? But, isn't that...*cold*?"

Focusing on inflammation control (rest, ice, protection, gentle exercise) for just five days can significantly change how you feel. So, if you don't like what you read here, go ahead and skip it. But if you're not making progress, come back to it, and try it for *just five days*.

A Perfect Day of Inflammation Management

- Use ice at least 2 times.
- Try various proven (proven means they work for you) rest positions throughout the day as you go about your normal activities.
- Use tools such as a lumbar corset, trekking poles, or walker to get around.
- Do the beginning exercises in the next chapter and use ice afterward.
- Avoid prolonged standing. If your hobby is cooking (or doing dishes), you smartly put a high stool in your kitchen so you can take breaks.
- When the legs feel weak, try not to push through it.

SUMMARY

Reducing swelling and inflammation in and around your spine:

- improves tissue health
- creates space for your spinal cord
- reduces symptoms of spinal stenosis

Inflammation control is an ongoing process. Good and bad days are a normal part of moving forward. Learning how your body responds to various self-management strategies, and implementing those that work best for you, is a great way to put yourself on the path to recovery.

ANTI-INFLAMMATORY EQUIPMENT LIST

- Soft Gel Ice Packs
- Elastic Lumbar Corset
- Front-wheel Walker
- Four-wheel Walker with Seat
- Cane
- Trekking Poles
- Kitchen Stool
- Recliner Chair
- Pillows, Bolsters, and Towel Rolls

- **DON'T**
    - Use ice over an area of numbness.
    - Use ice for more than 10 minutes.
    - Add more than one new activity or exercise in any given day.
    - Wear your lumbar corset 24 hours a day.
    - Let someone *push* (or *nag*) you into an upright position.
    - Start new exercises with 100% effort.

- **DO**
    - Use rest breaks and rest positions to reduce inflammation.
    - Use a walker or other device.
    - Use good body mechanics and a wide stance for bending activities.
    - Keep a list of things that aggravate your stenosis.
    - Use a lumbar corset to unload your spine.
    - Start new exercises using a minimum of effort.
    - Name a new puppy (if you want) "Inflammo."

Keep Moving with Strategic Exercise

< FOCUS AREA 2 >

INTRODUCTION

WHY KEEP MOVING?

Want to be healthy? Keep moving.

Movement improves the elasticity of your ligaments, and the health of your discs and bones. It stimulates blood flow and flushes toxins from the body. Movement, as opposed to sitting in one place for long periods, extends your life and decreases your chances of developing diabetes, heart disease, and cancer.

Movement is especially important for those of us with spinal stenosis. We need to do whatever we can to keep our ligaments healthy and supple, our capillary beds open and profuse, and our discs as hydrated as possible. Why? Because all these things can have an effect on how much room there is for our nerves and spinal cord. And because all these things slow the progression of degenerative joint disease in our spines. And, because we will feel better!

In recent years, a number of studies have suggested that sitting in one place for the majority of the day can be almost as bad for you as smoking. The more time someone spends sitting, the poorer his or her health. But for people with lumbar stenosis, to keep moving is not quite so easy. Stenosis symptoms are usually eased by sitting. There's a tendency to think, *Why not just sit here a little more? Heck, why not just sit here a lot more?*

Don't succumb! You can do it! All you need are a few good strategies. If walking short distances is all you can manage, then walk short distances frequently throughout the day. Walk for as long as you're comfortable, then supplement your program with an alternative to walking—such as pedaling a stationary bike or taking an aquatic exercise class.

WHAT'S THE BEST EXERCISE FOR SPINAL STENOSIS?

If only there *was* just one! Using sound principles of strategic exercise, I advise a combination of the following four categories:

- *Aerobic Exercise*
- *Stretching Hip Muscles*
- *Exercising Muscles that Attach to the Spine*
- *Loosening the Upper Back*

Including all of these elements in your spinal stenosis exercise program means you are *strategizing* to give yourself the best possible opportunity for improvement. Let's go into a little more detail on each of the four categories.

CATEGORY ONE: *Aerobic Exercise*

Low to moderate intensity sustained movement, aerobic exercise gets your heart pumping a little faster and your lungs working a little harder. Examples include: walking, jogging, cycling, rollerblading, and swimming. Current research indicates that regular aerobic exercise is one of the most important factors in determining whether a person with spinal stenosis can live relatively symptom-free. It is the most important aspect of your program, and hence it is the first one on the list.

CATEGORY TWO: *Stretching Hip Muscles*

Stretches are designed to increase the length and pliability of muscles. Just one tight hip muscle can wreak havoc on spinal stenosis. It does this by producing abnormal torque or tension in the spine and pelvis. When a tight hip muscle becomes loosened, it often becomes easier to stand up straight, get up from a chair, and take longer strides when walking.

CATEGORY THREE: *Exercising Muscles that Attach to the Spine*

When we exercise aerobically, we are improving our circulatory system and the health of all our tissues. When we strengthen muscles that specifically attach to the spine, we're not only strengthening muscles that support the spine, we're improving local blood flow into and around the spine. *All strengthening exercises are circulation enhancing exercises.* Working these muscles on a daily basis is like giving our spines a nice drink of water or a plate of nutrient-rich food. And you can do it in just a few seconds.

CATEGORY FOUR: *Loosening the Upper Back*

It sounds a little far-fetched, but you can reduce a lot of pressure on your low back just by loosening up your upper back. If your spine is stiff, when you turn side-to-side, there's going to be a lot of friction—a lot of friction, and a lot of force generated where the low back meets the base of your pelvis. When your upper spine is more flexible, that rotation or bend is shared equally through all the joints of the spine. You'll have less pressure on your lower back and reduce wear and tear.

Before I go into more detail on each of the four categories, let me go into a little more depth on what I mean by *strategic exercise.*

71

WHAT IS STRATEGIC EXERCISE?

Strategic exercise is smart exercise—exercise designed to provide the best chance for success. All you need to do is keep to a few basic principles: Choose just one or two exercises at a time and a realistic goal. Use gradual progression (just...go... slow). And—should you have a flare-up—make adjustments. Don't just ditch the whole program!

Let's take a look at the exercise strategies of Kyle and Bill:

Kyle is told by his doctor to exercise for his spinal stenosis and to "get out and walk." The next day, he hits the sidewalk! His goal is to walk 3 miles per day until he starts feeling better. He doesn't use any kind of cane or walker because, "That'll just make me weak!" At about 500 feet, his legs are wobbly, but he keeps on going, determined to meet his goal. Finally, his legs give out from under him. Undeterred, Kyle drags himself to his feet and continues his walk. Then, he falls and breaks his hip. (You see, he literally did hit the sidewalk!) For the next 8 weeks, the only exercise he gets is hobbling to the bathroom on a walker, sitting in his recliner, and tossing a tennis ball across the house for his miniature dachshund, Rudolf. "I guess the whole exercise thing is not going to work for me," he sighs.

Kyle is practicing *non-strategic exercise.*

Bill is told by his doctor to exercise for his spinal stenosis and to "get out and walk." He buys this book, reads it, and has an exercise epiphany. He picks 1-2 beginning exercises, does them gently, and then waits a few days to see if he's flared up. If he's not flared up, he puts a little more *oomph* into them, and adds a few more until he has 3-5 basic non-aggravating exercises.

At the same time, he initiates his walking program. He finds out his maximum walking distance is 500 feet. He starts walking three sets of 400 feet with sitting breaks in between. He gradually, over a period of weeks, increases either the number of sets or the distance walked, making sure he avoids any fatigue or cramping in his legs. He buys a set of walking sticks and finds he can walk 1000 feet comfortably.

Bill walks, then does his exercises, then uses ice on his low back in a position of comfort. He progresses his program gradually, and uses other types of aerobic exercise such as bicycling or using a Nu-step to improve his overall health. Over time, Bill's symptoms improve.

Bill is practicing *strategic exercise.*

STRATEGIC EXERCISE VS. NON-STRATEGIC EXERCISE

STRATEGIC	NON-STRATEGIC
Based on realistic self-assessment	Based on unrealistic self-assessment
Purposeful	Random, impulsive
Gradual progression	Overly ambitious
Safe	Dangerous
Informed	Uninformed
Feels good, rewarding	Punishing or "no pain, no gain" attitude
Multifaceted	Tries one thing, then quits
Patient and OPTIMISTIC	Easily discouraged and PESSIMISTIC

Strategic exercise? Easy as pie! Let's review the basic principles:

- Start with *a few* exercises at a time.
- Come up with a *realistic* goal.
- Use *gradual* progression.
- If you have a flare-up, *make adjustments*.
- *Never* just ditch the whole program!

Now that we've gone over some basic guidelines for your exercise program, it's time to get started on the four strategic categories.

CATEGORY ONE
AEROBIC EXERCISE

INTRODUCTION

Improved cardiovascular health leads to improved health of the spine. This includes increased capillary circulation to and around the spine, as well as

- Improved health of ligaments, bones, discs, and fascia
- Increased pain tolerance
- Reduced inflammation of tissues

For overall cardiac health, The American Heart Association recommends a goal of at least 150 minutes (i.e. two-and-a-half hours) per week of some kind of moderate aerobic exercise.

This is equivalent to 30 minutes per day for five days a week. Of course, if you're someone who's never exercised before or is not in condition, you should NOT immediately fling yourself into 30-minute workouts. It's a goal, not an ultimatum!

If you are just getting started with aerobic exercise, ease in with 10 minutes at a time. You can even begin with only three to five minutes at a time. It's perfectly acceptable to put in three ten-minute workouts daily. Even five three-minute workouts are better than zero!

SUMMARY OF AEROBIC EXERCISE GOALS

Beginning Level

5–10 minutes total
3–7 days per week

Intermediate Level

15–20 minutes total
3–7 days per week

Advanced Level

30–45 minutes total
3–5 days per week

*Always consult a trained healthcare professional before beginning any new exercise program.

SAFETY RECOMMENDATIONS

Among readers, I anticipate a wide range in individual health statuses. This section covers aerobic exercise in how it relates to spinal stenosis. It does not provide personalized advise on how to *safely* aerobic exercise. I strongly recommend that before beginning any new exercise program you should:

- Check with your healthcare provider regarding any exercise limitations you may have.
- Be able and prepared to monitor your own heart rate.
- Determine your safe target heart rate for achieving a moderate level of aerobic exercise.
- Know the warning signs for over-exertion, heart attack, and stroke.

For more helpful and comprehensive information on this topic, visit the web site of the American Heart Association: **www.heart.org**.

WALKING: BENEFITS AND PITFALLS

For most people, the easiest type of aerobic exercise is walking. There's no equipment needed and you can just sail out the door and go.

Unfortunately, aerobic level walking can be difficult for people with spinal stenosis. You may find your legs feeling heavy, weak, or rubbery the longer you're on your feet. You may have more leg or back pain. Some people get an uncomfortable heaviness or pressure at the base of the spine. These symptoms are often eased by sitting or bending forward. When you are having these types of symptoms, forcing yourself to "walk through it" is probably not going to help. As your legs feel weaker and weaker, you are at risk for falling. Find a place to sit down before this happens.

The solution to this problem is NOT to totally give up walking. Let's face it, all of us who *can* walk want to keep on being able to walk. We want to do our shopping, we want to go to church, to the movies. We want to go out with friends or go see a Tom Petty concert. We want to get around the house, and, at the very least, to be able to make it to the bathroom, right? So it doesn't make sense to decide to totally call it quits.

What I recommend is that you do *as much walking as you can,* but if you can't do *enough* to get that 150 minutes per week, it's better to try something else. This can include:

- Aerobic Alternatives to Walking
- Assisted Walking
- Shuttle Walking
- Various Combinations

> **Note:** If you're already getting some type of aerobic exercise, there's no need to modify your program—*unless you're having symptoms*. If your Zumba class or jogging club is working for you, why switch? Those who are athletic and have excellent balance should feel free to substitute more vigorous forms of exercise, such as rollerblading, skiing, or road biking.

AEROBIC ALTERNATIVES TO WALKING

These are ways you can still get aerobic exercise without being stuck on your feet. Because symptoms of stenosis are often alleviated by sitting, most of the things I'll be suggesting are done in a sitting position. Here's the great thing about this strategy: Even if you *only* focus on walking alternatives, you should still begin to see improvement in your ability to walk and stand for long periods.

ASSISTED WALKING

Assisted walking (which includes using trekking poles, or a treadmill, or some kind of walker or cane) is a strategy to help you stay on your feet longer. When you can stay on your feet longer, you can improve your aerobic conditioning level—and that's the main goal.

SHUTTLE WALKING

The definition of the word *shuttle* is to go back and forth between two points. Shuttle walking is a way to use the amount of walking you *can* do for maximum aerobic effort. For some people, this could be walking back and forth across the house, pausing to rest in a chair between trips. Others can simply plan a longer walk with multiple rest stops along the way.

VARIOUS COMBINATIONS

In many cases, a combination of many different types of aerobic exercise provides optimal results. I don't believe there is only one way to do something, and I encourage you to use the information in these pages to run your own little experiments, to discover through trial and error what works best for you.

AEROBIC ALTERNATIVES TO WALKING

If you are unable to walk more than 3 minutes, or even 5 or 20 minutes, why not supplement your aerobic exercise strategy with something other than walking?

The next several pages list, roughly from least to most difficult, some alternative exercises to walking best-suited to lumbar spinal stenosis. Choose the one that feels the best, and stick with it. Remember, everyone's case is different.

It's also OK to combine two or more of these different exercises (including a little walking) in one session. Your long-term goal is to get that 150 minutes per week.

IMPORTANT TO REMEMBER!

For overall cardiac health, The American Heart Association recommends a goal of *at least 150 minutes per week of some kind of moderate aerobic exercise.*

This is equivalent to 30 minutes per day for five days a week. Of course, if you're someone who's never exercised before or is not in condition, you should NOT immediately fling yourself into 30-minute workouts. It's a goal, not an ultimatum!

If you are just getting started with aerobic exercise, *ease in* with 10 minutes at a time. You may even need to begin with only 3–5 minutes at a time. It's perfectly acceptable to put in three ten-minute workouts—or walks—daily.

Even five three-minute workouts or walking sessions are better than zero.

The inexpensive *floor pedaler* requires very low energy expenditure and is a great piece of equipment for people with severe deconditioning or respiratory disease. Just plop this beauty down in front of a firm-but-comfy chair, slip your feet into the pedals and off you go. If you're not used to exercising, pedaling for 3-5 one-minute intervals with 30-second rest breaks are a good place to start. I also recommend having a healthcare professional assist you.

Advantages: 1) Lowest impact and effort level of any exercise equipment. 2) Dirt-cheap, usually less than 30 bucks.

Disadvantages: 1) Too easy for some people. 2) Sometimes a bit squeaky and can wear out fast. 3) The centerpiece, where the gears are hidden, heats up with use and can burn you if you're not careful. 4) Sometimes you have to take the straps off to get your whole foot on the pedal.

> Caution advised for people with peripheral neuropathy, paralysis, or drop foot. It may be difficult to keep your feet on the pedals. Consult a therapist before trying this equipment.

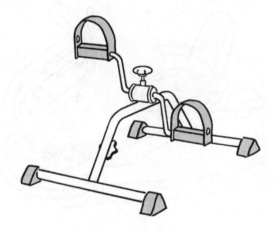

The squeaky wheel gets the grease.

The recumbent cross trainer (Nu-step) is a comfortable, easy-to-use cross between a recumbent bike and a stair master. The Nu-step provides the comfort of a recumbent bike without as much hip and knee movement. Its moveable arms and low stress on the joints makes it a great option for just about any ability level.

With its stable foot-plates, the Nu-step might just be the ideal piece of equipment for people with peripheral neuropathy. Even if you have numbness or weakness in your feet, the stable platform and stabilizer strap keeps them in place.

Use with or without the moveable arm attachments. If just starting out, use shortened movements in your legs, and hold your abs in to stabilize your hips.

Advantages: 1) Easy to use, low-impact aerobic workout in a stenosis-friendly position. 2) Many physical therapy clinics have these, so you can try them out with some supervision. 3) Very easy to climb onto, unlike some bikes or other equipment.

Disadvantages: 1) Going to set you back somewhere in the thousands for your own home model.

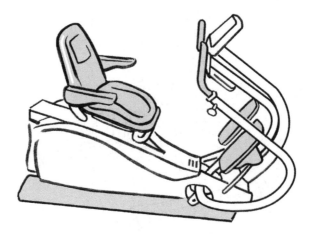

Try me. I'm fun!

I love upright stationary bikes! Because the pedals are almost directly below the pelvis, your feet circle happily beneath you, almost as if you are walking. Hang on to the handlebars, flexing your spine to relieve your stenosis symptoms. Or don't hang on to the handlebars, and get an aerobic workout while strengthening in an erect posture. (Or alternate between the two—it doesn't make you wishy-washy, it makes you smart!)

Advantages: 1) If your hips and knees are on the stiff side, it may be easier to pedal than a recumbent bike. 2) The closest thing to standing up you can do while still sitting. 3) Super easy to find cheap ones at garage sales or on craigslist.

Disadvantages: 1) Many of the seats for upright exercise bikes seem to have been designed by sadists. (When choosing an exercise bike, make sure you test out the seat. Or use padded bicycle shorts to minimize bun chafing.) 2) Some people just can't resist turning the tension on the bike up. This can cause aggravation of arthritic joints.

> Caution advised for people with peripheral neuropathy, paralysis, or drop foot. It may be difficult to keep your feet on the pedals. Consult a therapist before trying this equipment.

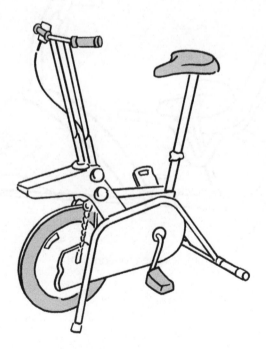

I'm the closest thing to walking that can still be called not walking!

Many people find a recumbent bike more comfortable than an upright bike. It's a little bit like climbing into an easy chair. With a recumbent bike, you have to be extra careful not to sit too far back from the pedals. Because the pedals are out in front of you — instead of directly under you — there is a risk of creating a pull on the sciatic nerve and hamstrings, which in turn puts torque on the spine. To avoid this, make sure your knees are a little bent at all times while pedaling.

Advantages: 1) Seat is more comfortable than upright bike. 2) Less tension in the neck and upper back.

Disadvantages: 1) May aggravate symptoms if you have the seat too far back. 2) Allows trunk muscles to relax while you exercise—you'll need an alternate exercise to strengthen them.

> Caution advised for people with peripheral neuropathy, paralysis, or drop foot. It may be difficult to keep your feet on the pedals. Consult a therapist before trying this equipment.

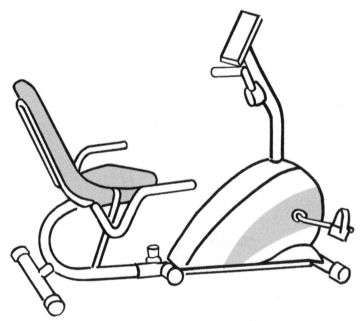

I'm designed for comfort!

ROWING MACHINE

Occasionally, clients ask me about rowing machines, and whether they can use them with spinal stenosis. I think rowing can be very advantageous, but advise proceeding with caution. As with any new type of exercise, it's best to try this one for a few minutes first, then progress from there in the following days. Start with small arcs of rowing before progressing yourself to larger ones.

Advantages: 1) Rowing specifically targets back muscles. 2) Can be tailored quite easily to fit your fitness and strength level. 3) Excellent for more fit individuals.

Disadvantages: 1) May involve large movements of hips and spine that will aggravate severe cases. 2) May not be comfortable for people with arthritic hips or knees.

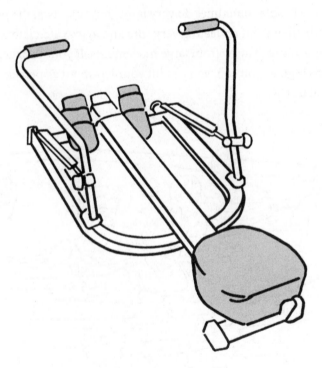

Row, row, row thyself.

Water exercise is a great way to get aerobic exercise that's easy on the joints. The water's built in resistance increases strength and endurance. Many people find it to be a very relaxing activity—especially if you just take some time to rest and float. You can also try conventional swimming or just walking back and forth across a pool.

Advantages: 1) Reduces compressive forces on the spine. 2) Can be tailored quite easily to fit your fitness and strength level. 3) A great way for overweight people to move easily and reduce pressure on the joints. 4) Provides a fun, social environment with friends to keep you motivated. 5) Gives you a chance to be supervised by an instructor while you exercise.

Disadvantages: 1) People sometimes do very large movements in the pool (it's easy and it feels good), then wind up feeling very sore and aggravated later. Avoid this pitfall by keeping yourself away from large movements. If your instructor tells you to lift your leg as high as you can, you can lift your leg about 25 percent as high as you can and still be OK.

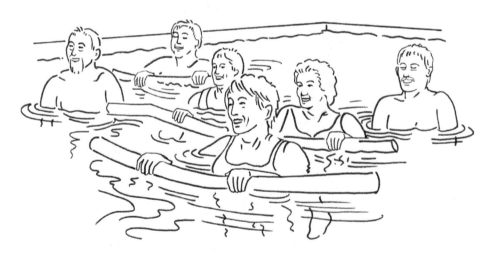

Water you waitin' for?

All the pain-creams, ointments, rubs, heating pads, and so on can't, in my experience, begin to do for a body what a simple thing like nature's water can do!
                                                                —Aunt Rose

Aunt Rose on Aquatic Exercise

"I love the pool. The water temp is kept at 92-94 degrees—well-treated and not over-powering. Even though I have a fear of water, the pool is well-equipped with safety devices and flotations to enable me to do my low impact exercises painlessly. The weightlessness I feel while exercising is encouraging and motivates me to continue. The ability to move parts of my body, already riddled with chronic pain, effortlessly, and get the same effect as I would get on dry land amazes me.

I would encourage all that have chronic pain to experience warm water therapy—as opposed to land therapy—as a means of keeping active.

Another perk is the comradery you build with others who are at the pool for the same reason. I'm working out my body and mind at the same time.

Every day I go, I'm a different person leaving than when I walked in.

I hope this encourages those who feel hopeless when it comes to exercise to realize there is hope.

Once I was terrified of water. Now, it's become my best friend!"

ASSISTED WALKING

Assisted walking is simply this: walking with the use of some kind of a device. These devices allow you to transfer some of your body weight through your arms to unload the spine. This helps you stay balanced, more upright, and on your feet longer. Assisted walking can also be used as an interim step to regular walking without a device.

Let's take a look at some of these devices and how they might work for you.

The front-wheel walker has two wheels in front and two plastic coasters in back, which are sometimes covered by tennis balls. If you're unable to walk 5 minutes without your legs feeling weak, painful, or cramped—see how it goes with a front-wheel walker.

Advantages: 1) Takes pressure off the spine. 2) More stable than a cane or 4-wheel walker (big plus!). 3) Great for "shuttle walking" (I'll explain later) on smooth, level surfaces.

Disadvantages: 1) It's slow. 2) There's no built-in seat. 3) Can be squeaky and parts wear out fast when you use them outside. 4) Difficult to propel on thick carpets. 5) You may have to conquer your discomfort with the stigma.

If you have a recent history of falls, feel like you could fall, or cannot tolerate walking 5 minutes or more, a front-wheel walker might be the ideal piece of *exercise* equipment for you. You'll also want to have someone along with you, just to be safe.

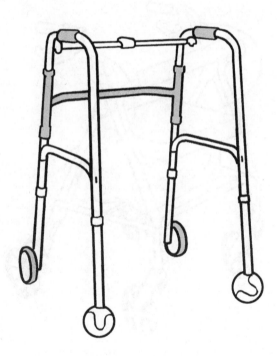

I'm stable.

Given a choice between a front-wheel walker and a four-wheel walker, who wouldn't choose the sportier four-wheel walker with built-in seat? Unfortunately, it does not unload the spine quite as much as the front-wheel walker, and is a little more difficult to handle.

Advantages: 1) Allows you to absorb *some* of the weight of your body through your arms. 2) Moves faster than the front-wheel walker, especially on sidewalks and other uneven surfaces, encouraging outdoor exercise. 3) Built-in seat for spontaneous rest breaks provides the freedom to get out and walk. 4) Smooth, noiseless ride. 5) Easier to propel on thick carpet. 6) Painted sports-car blue, gold, or red, these walkers look stylish.

Disadvantages: 1) Mostly provides just balance—if you try to put too much weight on the handles, it can slip out from under you. 2) Less easy to control the speed (though there are handbrakes), especially going down hills! 3) Not quite as stable as the front-wheel walker.

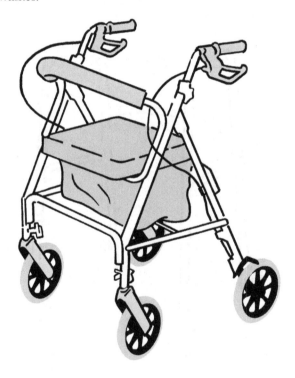

I'll give you more freedom!

Treadmills provide a more aerobic workout than most other exercise equipment. Many have adjustable inclines so you can simulate walking uphill (which makes you bend forward and is easier on your stenosis). My advice however is to not adjust the incline up more than a few levels (using too high of an incline can cause foot or tendon problems). If you tolerate walking 5 minutes without symptoms, the treadmill could be a good piece of equipment for you.

Advantages: 1) Handrails let you take some weight off the spine. 2) Possible to control pacing. 3) Easy to time yourself. 4) You can use it on a *slight* (no more than .5 to 1.0) incline—so you're always walking slightly uphill, and this takes pressure off the spine.

Disadvantages: 1) Fall risk. 2) Easy to overdo it. 3) Can be inconvenient to stop and take a sitting break.

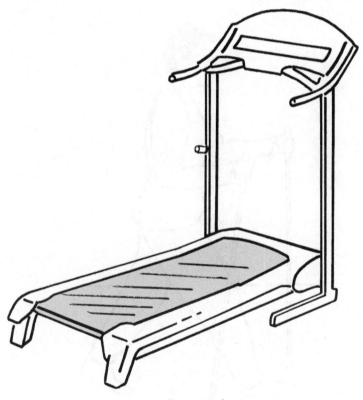

I'm sporty!

Trekking poles—also called "walking poles" or "walking sticks"—are a great alternative to using a walker outside. They also let enable you to go on soft dirt trails which reduce compressive forces on the spine. And they look really cool.

A perfectly good set of trekking poles is not hard to find. You can pick one up for about 30 bucks.

Advantages: 1) More supportive than a cane. 2) Fun to use on trails. 3) Feel good to use and get your upper body involved with the exercise.

Disadvantages: 1) Not as supportive as a walker. 2) Some people have trouble coordinating the movement. 3) Can be tripped over.

Trekking poles can be used a couple of different ways. Swing them forward in unison, driving them into the ground. Or alternate from one side to the other, like you're cross country skiing.

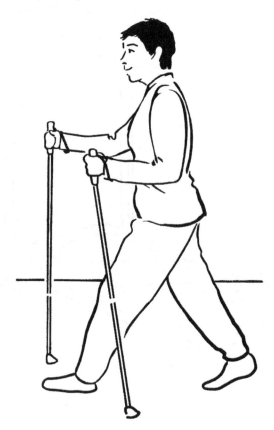

I look cool.

SHUTTLE WALKING

Many people with spinal stenosis feel immediate relief of their symptoms once they sit down. Because of this, you can stretch a 1 or 2 minute walk into a 5 or 10 minute walk by simply taking a sit-down break. Every 1-2 minutes, find a place to sit 30 seconds (longer if you need it) before you get up and walk again. To keep your aerobic workout going, use some exercise bands with your arms. This technique works best if you take that sit break *before* you start getting tired. First, test yourself to find out how far you can comfortably walk...then, just rest yourself before you get too close to that endpoint. Trial and error is the key to finding the perfect formula for you.

Shuttle walking can be used by both short and long distance walkers:

- *Beginning:* Every two hours: Walk back and forth across the house 2-3 times, using a wheeled walker, cane, trekking poles, or even nothing at all. Frequency trumps distance. Keep this up for 1-2 weeks until it becomes easy. If your legs feel weak after a single trip across the house, sit and rest for 30 seconds after each trip before starting the next one.
- *Intermediate Level:* Three times per day, walk 500 feet. Or try some two-minute stints on the treadmill or outside. Must have ability to sit and rest.
- *Advanced Level:* Use 5-10 minute walks with 1-2 minute sitting breaks to string together 10-30 minutes of aerobic exercise.

REVIEW

Although it is certainly possible to use walking as your primary exercise when you have spinal stenosis, you actually now have a number of options:

- You can do regular walking some of the time, assisted walking some of the time, and alternatives to walking some of the time.
- You can do all regular walking.
- You can do all assisted walking.
- You can do all alternatives to walking.
- You can do shuttle walking.
- You can do shuttle walking, supplemented by alternatives to walking.

All of the above choices, along with any other combos you can think of, will help you get the aerobic exercise you need to improve your overall health.

TIPS TO STAY ON YOUR FEET A LITTLE LONGER

1. *Wear supportive shoes.*
   A good walking or running shoe with an arch support that suits your foot can reduce compression and jarring of the spine. Protects knees, hips, ankles.

2. *Find softer terrain than concrete—gravel, dirt, or a rubberized running track.* Reduces compression and jarring of the spine. Protects knees, hips, ankles.

3. *Walk with an elastic lumbar corset.*
   Reduces pelvic movements that can sometimes aggravate stenosis.

4. *Use an assistive walking device—a cane, walker, or trekking poles.*
   Helps with balance, prevents falls, and takes weight off the spine.

5. *Try shuttle walking.*
   Recent evidence suggests small bursts of exercise followed by short rests in between can improve your cardiovascular health as well as traditional aerobic exercise. Several short walks with frequent sit-down breaks let you string together that winning combination.

6. *Get a walking buddy or join a group.*
   Walking companions motivate us and distract us from feeling tired.

STARTING A WALKING PROGRAM

Walking is the simplest form of aerobic exercise. Everyone enjoys mobility, but with spinal stenosis it can be daunting. I've outlined a simple test for identifying your level of walking ability. This can help you develop a walking program that works for you. It's also a great way to track your progress.

STEP ONE
Perform a Walking Self-Assessment

Figure out your Pre-Symptomatic Walking Time (PSWT) or Distance (PSWD). This is the amount of time (or distance) you can walk before you start to have symptoms. How to do it:

1. Time how long you can walk on level ground before you experience:

   - Discomfort, cramping, numbness, or weakness in the legs
   - A need to hunch over (more than when you started)
   - Any of the other symptoms (such as low back pain or aching) typically related to your spinal stenosis

2. Measure the distance walked before these symptoms kick in. You can be really specific (with a pedometer) or use a rough estimate ("I can walk to the mailbox and back.")

3. Write it down and track it, using your own system or the chart on page 94.

STEP TWO
Start Adding Variables to See If You Can Increase the Time on Your Feet

See if your PSWT or PSWD increases with the use of:

- A cane
- Trekking poles
- A four-wheeled walker with seat
- A treadmill
- A front-wheeled walker
- A lumbar corset

If your walking tolerance increases with one of the above, consider using it for your walking program. You don't have to try each and every one of them, but the more you experiment, the more information you'll have, and the better you'll be able to identify what works best for you.

TRACKING WALKABLE TIME AND DISTANCE
(SAMPLE CHARTS)

Date:	nothing	cane	poles	walker	treadmill	corset
PSWT **Pre-Symptomatic** **Walking Time** (seconds or minutes)						
PSWD **Pre-Symptomatic** **Walking Distance** (steps, feet, or destination)						

Date:	nothing	cane	poles	walker	treadmill	corset
PSWT **Pre-Symptomatic** **Walking Time** (seconds or minutes)						
PSWD **Pre-Symptomatic** **Walking Distance** (steps, feet, or destination)						

Date:	nothing	cane	poles	walker	treadmill	corset
PSWT **Pre-Symptomatic** **Walking Time** (seconds or minutes)						
PSWD **Pre-Symptomatic** **Walking Distance** (steps, feet, or destination)						

STEP THREE
Categorize and Strategize

See which of these categories is the best fit for you:

BRONZE BULLET

500 feet or less or less than 5 minutes.
In order to get 150 minutes per week of aerobic exercise, you'll need focus on alternatives to walking (exercise bicycle, pedaler, or Nu-step) while supplementing with some type of assisted walking (walker, 4-wheel walker, or trekking poles).

A good walking program strategy would be to *shuttle walk* a comfortable distance for you, with a 30-second seated rest in between. Continue to *shuttle walk* for 10–30 minutes or until your ability to walk half the distance of your PSWD becomes difficult.

Some of us begin at Bronze Bullet and stay there. This is perfectly respectable. This isn't a race or competition; this is about feeling the best you can feel.

SILVER TORPEDO

Able to walk between 500 and 999 feet or between 5 and 15 minutes.
To reach your goal of 150 minutes per week, you can walk 10–15 minutes twice daily for five days per week. You may want to supplement this with longer sessions of an alternate type of exercise, like water aerobics or an exercise bicycle. You can also extend your walking time using trekking poles or a treadmill.

GOLDEN CHARIOT (AKA PLATINUM GRAND POOBAH)

Able to walk more than 1000 feet and more than 15 minutes.
You can probably use walking as your primary aerobic exercise and still achieve your 150 minute per week goal. You might incorporate trekking poles into longer walks, use a treadmill, or use another type of alternative exercise to get your heart rate up a little higher, or to just get some variety.

OK — Now What?

Now that you've found your category, use the strategy associated with it to see if you can

1. Improve your pre-symptomatic walking time (PSWT) or distance (PSWD).
2. Meet the criteria of 150 minutes per week of moderate aerobic exercise.
3. Make yourself feel better gradually over time.

SUMMARY

- Improved cardiovascular health leads to improved health of the spine.
- For overall cardiac health, The American Heart Association recommends a goal of at least 150 minutes (i.e. two-and-a-half hours) per week of some kind of moderate aerobic exercise.
- Always consult a trained healthcare professional before beginning any new exercise program.
- Walking is not the only way you can get aerobic exercise.
- Assistive devices allow you to unload the spine. This lets you stay on your feet a bit longer.
- Shuttle walking can be used by both short and long distance walkers.
- A combination of many different types of aerobic exercise provides optimal results.

CATEGORY TWO
STRETCHING HIP MUSCLES

INTRODUCTION TO STRETCHING

In my experience, when stenosis patients get flared up from exercising, the stretches are often to blame. Not because stretching is bad, but because it can be a little tricky when you have spinal stenosis. Remember, you've got limited space for the nerves and spinal cord. If you overdo the stretch, the spine gets torqued and you can pinch or irritate a very sensitive nerve. It's a natural impulse to go for the gusto, even when it hurts a little, but—trust me—you're better off taking it easy with stretches.

Exercises are sometimes hard to learn from a diagram. To help you with some of the finer points, I've posted videos of each exercise which are free for you or anyone to watch on **www.rehabspinalstenosis.com**.

STRETCHING TIPS TO KEEP YOU ON TRACK

- *Go for a subtle pull, not a strong one*. More is NOT better.
- *Hold your stretch for 30 seconds*. If your stretch starts to bother you, release the tension a little and continue holding.
- *Take deep, relaxing breaths*. As you exhale, focus on relaxing the muscle you are stretching.
- *Keep your pelvis stable*. When stretching hip muscles, keep your pelvis from rotating and your spine from flexing too much one way or the other.
- *Wear loose-fitting clothing*.
- *Don't feel obligated to do stretches on the floor*. You can do them on the bed. It's fine.
- *Give yourself a five- to ten-minute warm-up with some type of aerobic exercise*.

Avoid any kind of over-vigorous stretching. Keep things subtle and you'll do great!

Just one tight hip muscle can wreak havoc on spinal stenosis, and it's important to take care of this if it's a problem for you. Hip muscle tightness limits the mobility of the pelvis. This forces your spine to take on extra work. The following stretching exercises are listed from easiest to most difficult, and should be added to your program one at a time—waiting at least 2-3 days after each new exercise (just to make sure you're OK) before adding a new one. Please visit **www.rehabspinalstenosis. com** for video tips on doing these stretches safely. The videos will also show you alternate ways to do the exercise that might be more effective for you.

Single Knee to Chest (30 seconds each leg × 2)

This one's so easy, I call it a "gimme" exercise. Lie on your back with your knees bent as shown. Slowly, lift one leg, keeping the knee bent. Place your hands behind your knee and pull toward your chest. When you feel a slight stretch, stop, and hold for 30 seconds. As you're holding, take deep breaths. Every time you exhale, focus on relaxing both your back and buttock muscles. If you're feeling sore, this is a great exercise to start with. It's also a great one to finish with, because it usually feels good.

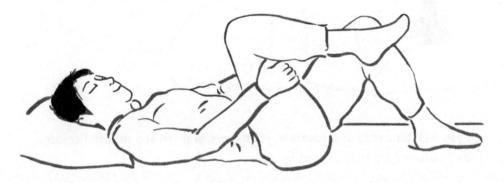

Once you do this exercise a few days in a row and are not feeling sore from it, you can try adding the "Double Knee to Chest" stretch, described on the next page.

Double Knee to Chest (30 seconds × 2)

First bring one knee up and hold, then slowly bring the other knee up and hold. Take a deep breath, and as you exhale, focus on relaxing your hips and keeping your back in contact with the bed or mat.

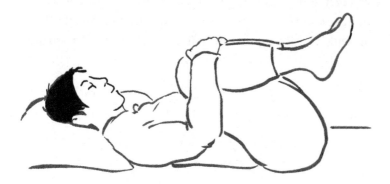

If you feel some pain or pressure in your knees, you can accomplish the same thing by pulling from behind your knees:

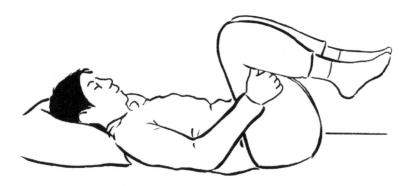

What's with all the breathing during these exercises? Deep breathing promotes relaxation and allows for a better stretch. It also helps increase the supply of oxygen to your tissues.

Diagonal Knee to Chest Stretch (30 seconds each leg × 2)

This stretch focuses on an oft-tight hip muscle called the *gluteus medius*. Lying on your back, bring one knee up as if you're going to pull it to your chest. Instead pull the knee across your body. DO NOT allow your pelvis to rotate with this movement. You should feel the stretch somewhere around the side of your hip or buttock. Go for a light, comfortable stretch. Breathe deeply, relax your hip muscles as you exhale.

- The pull is felt to the outside of your buttock—not the groin
- Do not let your pelvis rotate along with the movement
- The direction of the stretch should not be at a sharp angle.
- Your spine should not twist—keep low back in contact with the exercise surface

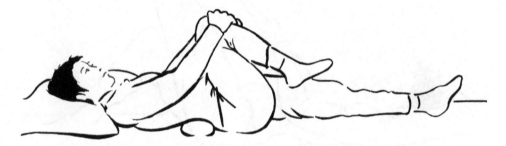

Here's another view:

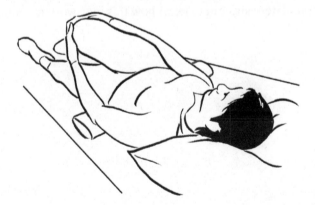

The model is using a towel roll to remind her to keep her spine from twisting. Watch the video at **www.rehabspinalstenosis.com** to learn how this may work for you.

Hamstring Stretch (30 seconds each leg × 2)

Lie on your back with one knee bent up. Using a long strap, belt, towel, or rope, pull your other leg up straight (or with the knee just slightly bent) until you feel a gentle pull. Hold 30 seconds. Please, make sure you start *very gently* and give yourself a few days to make sure you're doing OK.

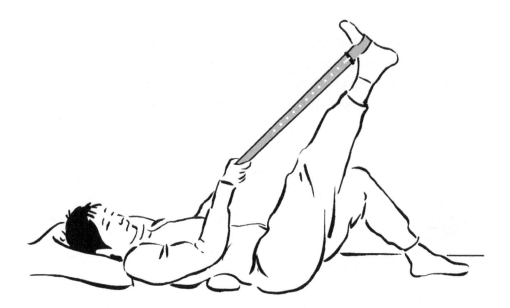

Our model uses a towel roll to keep her spine secure and stable. Watch the video at **www.rehabspinalstenosis.com** to learn how this may work for you.

Prone Knee Bend (2 seconds on each leg × 10)

If you felt the "Diagonal Knee to Chest" stretch in your groin instead of your hip, you might just have tight thigh muscles. Stretching these muscles can help you stand up straighter with fewer symptoms.

Lie face-down with a pillow under your stomach. Keeping your back flat, slowly bend one knee until you feel a *mild* stretch in the *front of your thigh*. Hold for a few seconds, then slowly lower. Repeat 10 times each leg. If your low back arches during this exercise, you are doing it incorrectly. Tightening your abs and buttocks during the movement helps keep the pelvis stable so you feel the stretch just a little sooner—that's good. You want to look something like this:

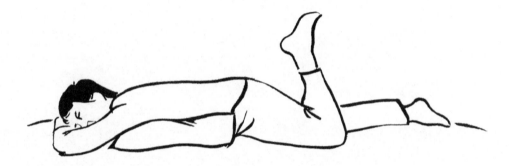

If you feel the pull in your low back or get a cramp in the back of your leg, you are not doing it quite right. Your back may be arching like this:

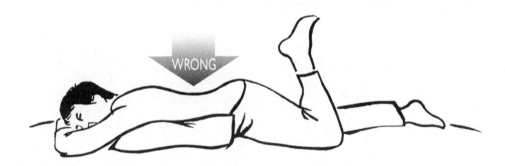

This stretch is considered advanced because it is difficult to do correctly. The holds are shorter because it takes a little effort. It might be a good idea to have a physical therapist help. For a video, go to **www.rehabspinalstenosis.com**.

SUMMARY POINTS

- Tight hip muscles can aggravate the symptoms of stenosis.
- A five- to ten-minute light aerobic warm-up is a good idea before stretching.
- Stretches should be more subtle than vigorous and include deep breathing.
- Avoid twisting or creating too much torque on the spine.
- After adding a new stretch, always wait a few days to make sure you feel OK.

CATEGORY THREE
EXERCISING MUSCLES THAT ATTACH TO THE SPINE

Assume the exercises in this section are going to make you feel better. They're going to enable you to walk a little bit farther, move more easily, and improve your balance. You'll notice it's easier to get in and out of bed.

Some of the exercises cited are quite simple. You can do them effectively without much fine tuning. Some of them are more complicated, or will be more effective with some extra help. Due to the limits of what a drawing can accomplish, I've posted videos of all of the exercises on **www.rehabspinalstenosis.com**.

WHY STRENGTHEN?

Physical therapists and athletic trainers are well-versed in ways to strengthen different muscles. You may be told by these professionals that certain muscles need to be stronger to *support* certain injured joints. If you have strong leg muscles or butt muscles, your knee will be well-supported. If you have strong abs or back muscles, your spine will be more stable. This is the conventional way we think of exercise: Your spine is a ship mast, supported by ropes and pulleys (muscles). Strengthen the ropes and pulleys and your spine will be better supported. Well, to some degree, this is true. But this is by no means the only reason to do—or way to think of—strengthening.

First of all, let me state the obvious: Your spine may be *like* a ship mast, but it is not a ship mast. (Nor is it a stack of Krispy Kreme donuts.) When we think of the spine as a ship mast, it helps us to understand muscles from a mechanical perspective. But at the same time, it helps us to *not* understand muscles. How so?

Ropes, pulleys, and ship masts are not alive. Muscles, ligaments, discs, nerves, and bones are. Ropes, pulleys, and ship masts don't have a blood supply. Ropes, pulleys and ship masts aren't *interconnected* by blood vessel networks (circulation), moist elastic cobwebs (fascia), and the exchange of fluids through cells (perfusion). Muscles, ligaments, discs, nerves, and bones are.

To understand muscles, ligaments, discs, nerves, and bones, we have to think like a physiologist. Things like joint lubrication, circulation, and tissue pliability become just as important as force, direction, and torque.

So, how can we use strengthening exercises for maximum benefit?

- *Use strengthening to MOVE stronger.* Focus on improving the strength of *movements* rather than one individual muscle. Having strong ropes and pulleys (muscles) helps, but strengthening one uber-important muscle won't work. Why? Because there isn't one uber-important muscle.
- *Use strengthening to improve the health of the body's tissue.* This includes bones, tendons, ligaments, fascia, muscles, blood vessels, and nerves. Strength exercises improve circulation, metabolism, nutrition, suppleness, and hydration. They help inflammation zones to become un-inflamed, hardened tissue or scarred tissue to become soft, and starved or thirsty tissue to become nourished and hydrated. For this reason, targeting muscles that attach to the spine improves the overall health of all the tissues of the spine.

HOW MANY REPETITIONS ARE ENOUGH?

You may need only 2-3 repetitions ("reps") of an exercise to get stronger, but your goal is not to have a single burst of strength—it's to be strong for the long haul. Do you want to be able to take a single strong step or several strong steps? For the purposes of endurance: the more reps the better. To improve circulation, the more reps the better. I like 20, but have had clients who do more.

If the inability to be on your feet for long periods makes it difficult for you to get traditional aerobic exercise, and you don't have immediate access to alternative types of equipment, you can use multiple sets of various mat exercises (such as the ones listed in the next pages), using lots of repetitions to create a self-styled aerobic workout. Just like with shuttle walking, small bursts of exercise followed by short rests in between can improve your cardiovascular conditioning almost as well as traditional aerobic exercise.

POSITIONING YOURSELF TO EXERCISE

Many of the exercises in this section can be done lying down. This prevents a lot of movement in the spine that can sometimes cause a flare-up.

Fairly regularly, a client will report to me that she (or he) did not do her (or his) exercises because it's just too difficult to get down on the floor. This still takes me by surprise because I never specifically advise people to get down on the floor to exercise.

So, I want to make this clear: *You do not have to lie down on the floor.* Sure, you *can* lie on the floor, if that feels good to you. (Or if you just like the view.) You can also lie on a bed or even recline in a recliner. Some people like the firm surface of the floor, but it is not important at all. If you have difficulty getting down on the floor, I especially encourage you to avoid it because if you are uncontrolled in how you lower yourself to the floor, this may be aggravating to your symptoms.

Any exercise in this section can be modified in terms of position. The videos on **www.rehabspinalstenosis.com** provide some additional options that are not explained in this section.

Abdominal "Ab" Sets

Most people, when they think of abs, think of having a good six pack. But the "six pack" (it's actually an 8-pack) is only one of the abdominal muscles—the *rectus abdominis,* which is the most superficial of all of them. (It's the pretty one!) And while the rectus may provide some support to your spine, it does not even directly attach to your spine; it runs up and down from your pelvis to your ribs.

The *transverse abdominis* is the deepest of the ab muscles. It wraps around the torso like a muscular lumbar corset.

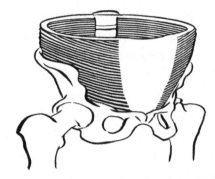

The *transverse abdominis* (along with two other deep abdominal muscles) also attaches to a large membranous sheath called the *thoracolumbar fascia*. Why care? Because the *thoracolumbar fascia* is intrinsic to the spine. It attaches to all the low lumbar spine bones and encases the muscles supporting the low back. This phenomenal diamond-shaped swatch also connects to deep spinal ligaments.

Take a look:

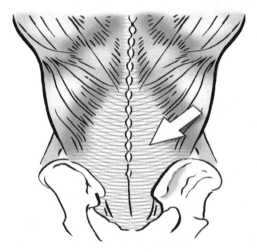

Thoracolumbar Fascia

Yes, the muscles connected to the thoracolumbar fascia form—among other things—a sort of corset. But exercising these muscles doesn't just help support the spine, it helps deliver nutrients to the spine. When you exercise to create tension in the thoracolumbar fascia, that tension, or, better, that combination of repeated contracting and relaxing (wringing out and opening, wringing out and opening) acts to pump blood into the area—like the pumping of a heart.

The other great thing about exercising the transverse abdominis is that when you contract it, there are other deep spinal muscles that contract along with it.

Remember to check **www.rehabspinalstenosis.com** for videos of these exercises.

Ab Set (GOAL: 20 reps)

Lie comfortably on your back with your knees bent, feet flat. You may need to lie in a slightly reclined position, such as in a recliner or on a bed with three or four pillows under your upper body. Or you may find it helpful to place your feet on a slight wedge. Once you've found a comfortable position, breathe deeply, and *relax*. Place your hands just above your pubic bone, on your lower abdominal muscles. Suck in your stomach like you would if you were trying to zip up a tight pair of jeans. Help it along with your hands as shown in the diagram—just a little scooping motion. Hold five seconds. (Keep breathing!) Then slowly release, and rest for five seconds. Start with 5 reps, twice daily. Over the next few weeks, work up to 20 reps all at once.

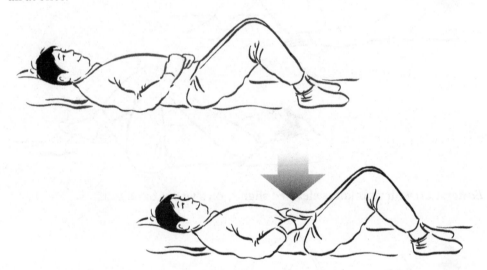

As your abdominals become stronger, you won't need to help with your hands so much. Just keep them lightly on your lower abdomen, so you can still feel the contraction of your muscles.

As your abs contract, you may feel a slight flattening of your back against the surface you're lying on. This is an unnecessary part of the exercise, but if it happens go ahead and let it—especially if it doesn't hurt. What I don't want you to do is *focus* on squeezing your buns together to tilt your hips back. This is what's known as a *substitution*—you're simply substituting your butt muscles for your abdominal muscles. So while you're doing this exercise, make sure you're feeling something happen in your abs.

Ab Set with Resist to Knee (GOAL: 20 reps)

Lie on your back with knees bent. Simultaneously flex your right hip and pull your abs in. Your knee comes up to the position in the picture. Then as you focus on tensing your abs, gently push your hand against your knee, and your knee against your hand, creating a bit of slight tension and hold in place. Hold 1–2–3, and slowly release. Do all repetitions on one leg before moving on to the other leg. Do not alternate. Start with 5 to 10 reps.

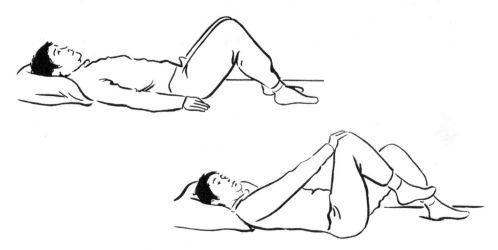

Easier: start with your knees elevated slightly on a wedge or bolster...

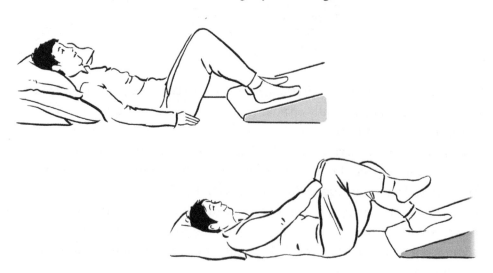

   I like this exercise a lot because you can really feel things working in there. It also seems to take a bit of pressure off the spine. I can feel my spine unloading each time I push my knee against my hand.

Seated Knee Lifts on Ball (GOAL: 20 reps)

Sit balanced on a 24-inch anti-burst gymnastic ball. (You can find one in the Sporting section of pretty much any department store). Feet about shoulder-width apart. Flex abs (pull in) as you lift one knee while maintaining your balance on the ball. Repeat with one leg 10 to 20 times until you can do it smoothly and consistently without losing your balance. Then you can try alternating legs. Note: Using a ball does not stress your abs any more than if you were doing it on a stable surface, like a chair. But it does require you to use your abs and legs together and *improve your balance.* (WARNING: This exercise can be a little tough, and I don't recommend it for anyone who is still in severe pain. Especially if you don't yet have the balance to do it without a lot of wobbling. In that case, you might try this sitting on a dining room chair).

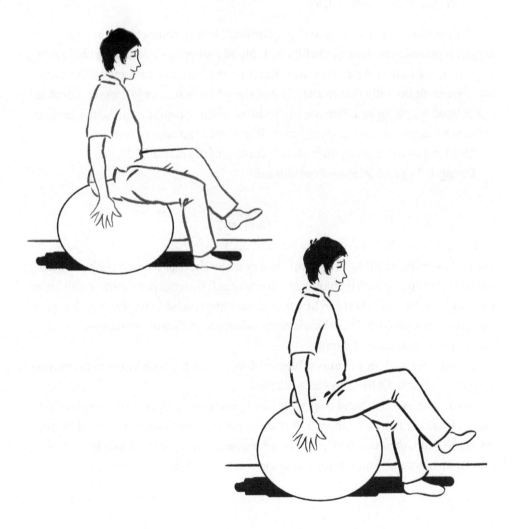

Latissimus "Lat" Pull

The *latissimus dorsi* (or "lat," as it is lovingly known by its friends) is the broadest muscle in your back, attaching to all the bones in the low back, half the bones of the upper back, the lower 3–4 ribs, your pelvic bones, your tailbone, the lower part of your shoulder blades, and various abdominal muscles. In the low back, the muscle merges with the *thoracolumbar fascia.*

Strengthening the lats and abs together is great for spinal stenosis. Together they form much of the body's natural muscular corset. But they also connect with the deeper structures of the spine that can benefit from increased blood flow. Blood flow is crucial to:

- reduce inflammation
- improve ligament elasticity
- hydrate intervertebral discs

Body builders do a lot of reps ("get pumped") before competing. They lift a weight repeatedly, so the muscle fills with blood and grows larger. This obviously impresses the judges. And that's the point. But, they are also improving the circulatory system of not only that muscle, but of the joints that muscle crosses. Consider that a good warm-up can increase the number of open capillary beds in a particular area by as much as a hundred times. That's one thousand percent!

This is what we're going for with our version of the *lat pull*.

Strength, but also *improved circulation*.

BEGINNING

Lat Pull with Ab Set (GOAL: 3 sets of 20)

For this exercise, you'll need to invest in a stretchy sheet of colored rubber called an exercise band. (Exercise bands are pretty much the cheapest home gym I know. I totally love the stuff!) You can buy it at almost any medical supply store, but you can also find it on-line. These bands come in several different resistances. You'll need a piece about 4–6 feet long.

Lie on your back in a comfortable position, preferably with knees bent, maybe your head elevated a little on some pillows.

Secure the exercise band over your head, as shown in the illustration. You can have a friend or family member stand at the head of the bed (or recliner) holding on to the band, or you can loop it around something sturdy, such as a hook or a pole or an elephant. Sometimes a bedpost works — as long as it's sturdy.

If you are a beginner, you'll want to start with an easier color level of exercise band. Don't worry if the exercise doesn't feel difficult. Once you crank out three sets of 20 reps, you'll be able to evaluate over the next few days whether you actually got a workout or not.

Grasp each end of the band (If you have arthritis in your hands or wrists, you may want to tie some loops into the ends of the band, or invest in some awesome attachable handles), keeping your elbows slightly bent (about 10°) and pulling your abs in at the same time (do an ab set!), pull down and OUT (without bending your elbows!). You should feel a tightening in your abs and back.

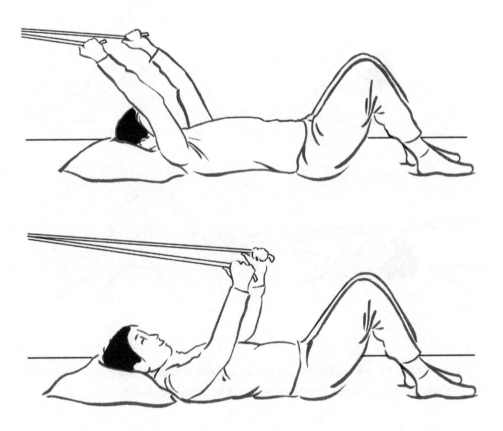

Start with about 10 reps, and do three sets. Before you move up to a more difficult color of exercise band, you should be able to do three sets of 20 without feeling sore the next day.

For video instructions go to **www.rehabspinalstenosis.com**. I'll go over some of the finer points of this exercise not covered by the book.

Lat Pull with Ab Set (Increased Vigor, Arc Distance, and Speed)
(GOAL: 3 × 20)

Perform the exercise as described on the previous page. This time, increase the length of the arc, increase the tension on the band (or get a stronger band), or increase the speed. And increase the reps to 3 sets of 20.

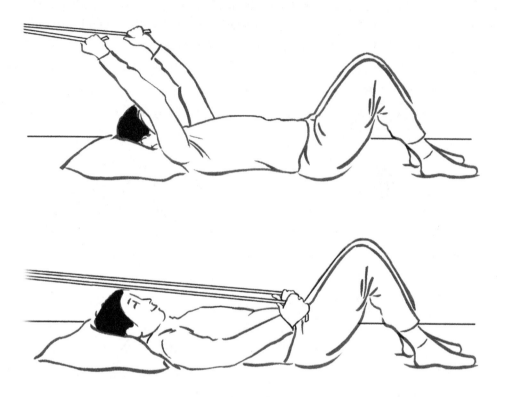

If you want to get a kind of aerobic workout from this exercise, increase your reps to 5 sets of 20. Just make sure you progress yourself gradually.

Standing Lat Pull with Ab Set (GOAL: 3 × 20)

Stand with a long piece of exercise band draped over a standard door. Stand in front of the edge of the door with your feet wider than shoulder-width apart. Keep the knees slightly flexed. Pull your abs in and do a slight pelvic tilt, so your low back flattens. Stand as close to the door as possible, and place your forehead gently against it. This keeps the door from swinging, and protects your eyes if the band happens to break. Perform the "Lat Pull with Ab Set" just as if you were doing it lying down. Remember not to use your elbows. The movement comes from your shoulder blades and shoulders.

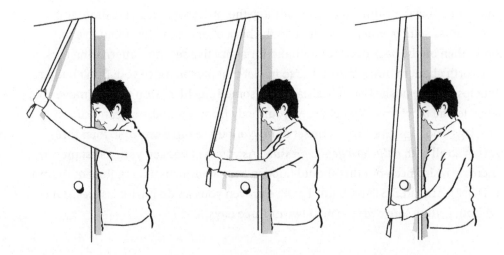

Just as with the beginning and intermediate lat pull (performed lying down), the standing lat pull can use short or long arcs of movement, with more or less tension on the band. Go to **www.rehabspinalstenosis.com** to watch a video of this exercise.

Resisted Trunk Rotation

This exercise wakes up the abs, hips, and legs, but also some deeper spine-stabilizing muscles. Remember, the goal of these exercises is not just to strengthen, but to shunt blood to the areas of your spine that need it most.

BEGINNING

Resisted Trunk Rotation (GOAL: 3 sets of 10)

This exercise requires the assistance of another person, someone you trust to be gentle.

Lie comfortably on your back with your knees bent, feet flat. As shown in the diagram, place the palms of your hands together in a prayer type position. Your exercise assistant *gently* pushes first on the back of one hand for about five seconds, then on the back of the other hand for about five seconds, alternating back and forth about 10 times. Your job is to not let that person move you. Don't budge! It helps if, as he pushes, your assistant says something like, "Don't let me move you, don't let me move you." To help keep your body from rotating, you can use your abs, legs, and hips. Start with one set of 10. Work up to three sets of 10 then three sets of 20 all with *only very gentle pressure*. As you get stronger, your assistant can increase resistance—but this should happen over a number of days. Rule of thumb is DON'T ADD RESISTANCE until you've proven you can do it with less resistance without getting sore over the next two or three days.

For video instructions go to **www.rehabspinalstenosis.com**

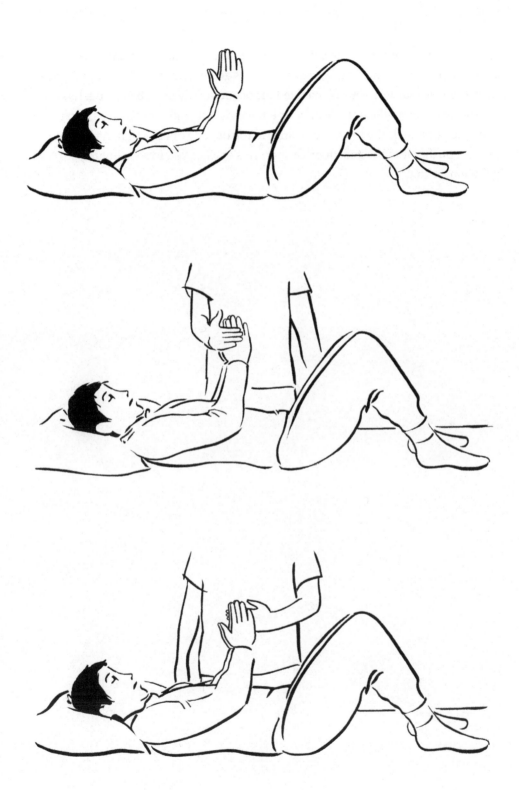

Resisted Trunk Rotation (Increased Vigor)
(GOAL: 3 sets of 10)

Same exercise, more resistance. If your shoulders are healthy, you can bring your arms up 90 degrees. In this way, more torque is generated through the arms. You may also feel your legs getting involved more—definitely not a bad thing. If the resistance comes to the outside of your left hand, your right foot pushes into the bed, floor, or mat. If the resistance comes to the outside of your right hand, your left foot pushes into the bed, floor, or mat. This teaches you to coordinate your legs with your trunk.

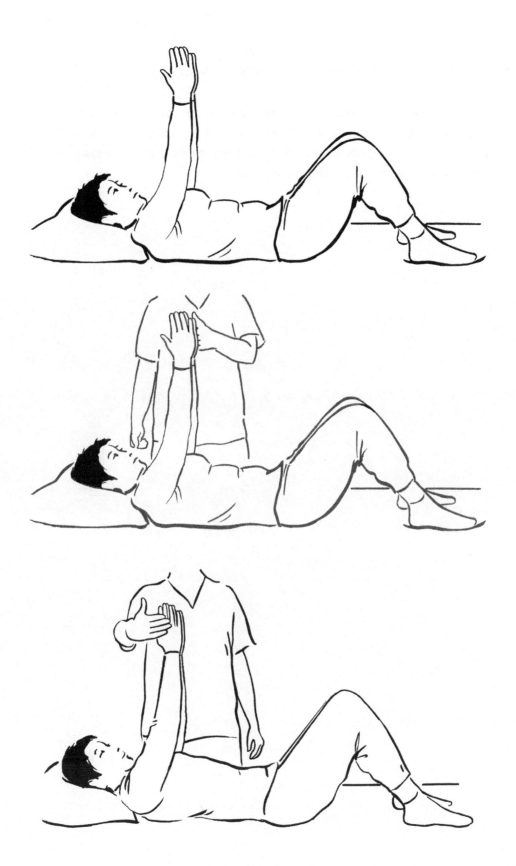

Resisted Trunk Rotation (shoulders flexed 100 degrees)
(GOAL: 3 sets of 20)

Just as bringing your arms up straight increases the difficulty of this exercise. If you flex your shoulders even more...presto! You get more difficulty. I like adding this degree of difficulty even if it's only for 3–5 reps because you have to learn to work your muscles in a more elongated position.

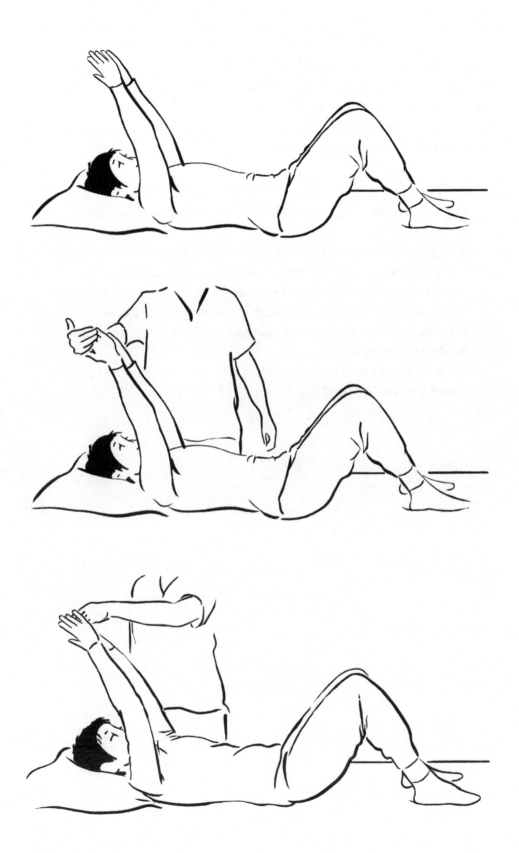

OTHER STRENGTHENING EXERCISES

Are there other good strengthening exercises for spinal stenosis? Sure, there are! Lots of them! The ones included here are just a few I've found to be the safest, most effective, and the least likely to flare you up. For a winning combination: stick to the one-new-exercise-at-a-time plan and progress yourself slowly. Remember, it's your body, and you're in the driver's seat.

SUMMARY

- Targeted strengthening can improve blood flow to muscles, ligaments, tendons, and fascia.
- Strength exercises can improve the patterning and control of our movements.
- Strength exercises can improve muscular support for the spine.
- The *transverse abdominis* is the deepest of the ab muscles and attaches to deeper structures of the spine through the thoracolumbar fascia.
- The *latissimus dorsi* also attaches to deeper structures of the spine through the thoracolumbar fascia.
- Adequate blood flow is crucial to reduce inflammation, improve ligament elasticity, and to hydrate discs.

CATEGORY FOUR
LOOSENING THE UPPER BACK

SELF-MOBILIZATION AND YOU

George has been hiking around Seattle's Lincoln Park every morning for the past 30 years. He gets there right at the crack of dawn, loves the chatter of birds and squirrels, breathes in the fresh air, and feels invigorated for the rest of the day.

Now that he's 67, though, George's knees are a little stiff, especially the right one. When he first starts out, he gets a sharp pain under his kneecap. This makes him limp a bit, but George has figured out a way to keep going. After a few minutes, he stops on the trail, bends and straightens his knee about twenty times vigorously, and is good to go from there. His sharp pain is gone! George is performing a "self-mobilization."

Self-mobilization refers to repeated movement of a joint or joints to increase joint lubrication, limber up ligaments, and relax surrounding muscles. In short, a quick way to loosen up a joint so it works better!

WHY LOOSEN THE UPPER BACK?

You're lost in the woods and you want to start a fire. What do you do? You might try striking two rocks together to get a spark. Or you might try spinning a very straight stick into some dry leaves placed on a rock. The spinning of the stick creates friction, and friction creates heat—in this case, the building heat needed to start the fire. Now, you're spinning and spinning the stick—does the whole stick get hot? No, of course not! Just the part at the bottom, where it twists against the rock. Well, what if the stick is really flexible and green? What if the stick twists around on itself like a spring? Well, then you can pretty much twist all you want. A flexible stick just doesn't generate enough heat to light a fire.

Now, imagine your spine is the stick. If your spine is stiff, when you turn side-to-side, well, right at the bottom lumbar bone over the base of your pelvis, there's going to be a lot of friction— a lot of friction, a lot of force, and a lot of wear and tear. Your low lumbar disc gets hot and inflamed.

Now, imagine your spine is like a green stick, a twisty stick, like a spring. Suddenly, instead of the rotation concentrating at the base of your spine, it's shared equally throughout the spine.

Now, *I don't want to* start a fire at the base of my spine.

I want the spine like the spring.

There are many types of exercises to loosen the upper back. For the purposes of this book, I'll list just a few very gentle self-mobilizations you can do with a simple towel roll. Techniques are listed from easiest to most difficult. You'll need to make sure you're comfortable while you do them.

For video instructions, go to **www.rehabspinalstenosis.com.**

Towel Roll Exercise to Loosen the Upper Back #1
(GOAL: 10 minutes)

This might just be the easiest exercise in the world! All you have to do is relax and take deep breaths.

Find a towel and roll it up. Lie on your back with the towel extending the entire length of your *upper back only*. The towel should be centered right between your shoulder blades. Next, just relax, and let your shoulders fall back. Take a deep breath. Breathe in, in, in. Feel your chest rise. Exhale, and just...relax. After 10 deep breaths, continue lying on the towel, taking normal breaths and relaxing for 5–10 minutes.

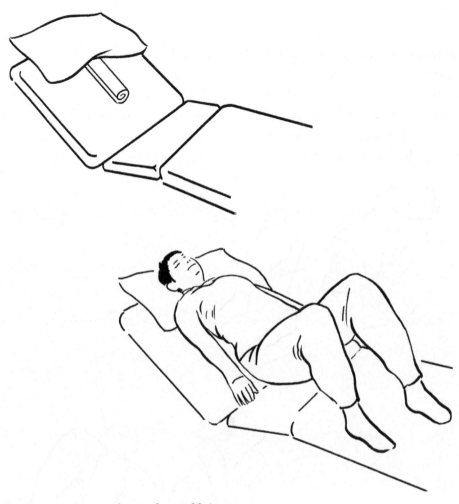

This exercise can be performed lying:

- flat on your back.
- flat on your back with knees bent.
- with your upper back propped on pillows.
- with your upper back propped on pillows and a pillow under your knees
- in a recliner

Feel free to try this with different-sized towel rolls: The smaller the more comfortable, the larger the better the stretch. Remember, the position *should not be painful.*

Towel Roll Exercise to Loosen the Upper Back #2
(GOAL: 10–20 repetitions)

The version just brings a little more motion into the picture. Lie on your towel roll as described on the previous page. Place your hands at your sides (you may find this more comfortable if you prop them up on pillows). Take a deep breath. Breathe in, in, in...as you *roll your palms up, squeeze your shoulders back, and stick out your chest.* Now, breathe out, and relax. Relax your chest, your shoulders. Let your palms roll down. Start with 5 to 10 reps.

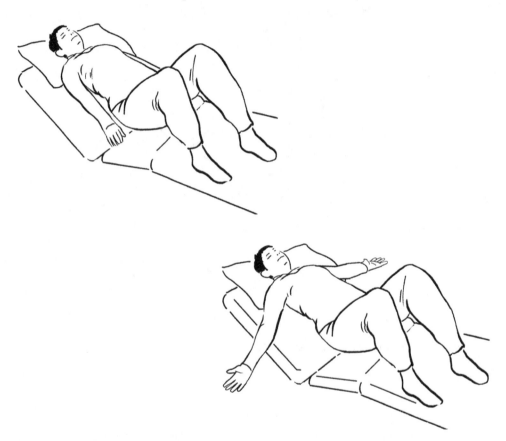

Towel Roll Exercise to Loosen the Upper Back #3
(GOAL: 10–20 repetitions)

Here's where we attempt to move the upper back like a spring. Lie on your towel roll as described earlier. Place your hands a small way out from your sides (you can prop your arms on pillows, if you need to, for comfort). As you lie on the towel, breathe in. As you breathe out, reach to one side, so your body glides and rotates sideways over the towel roll. Breathe in again, and return to center. Repeat this movement from side-to-side. For best results, try this exercise with your arms out 45, 60, and 90 degrees. See which angle feels best or stretchiest.

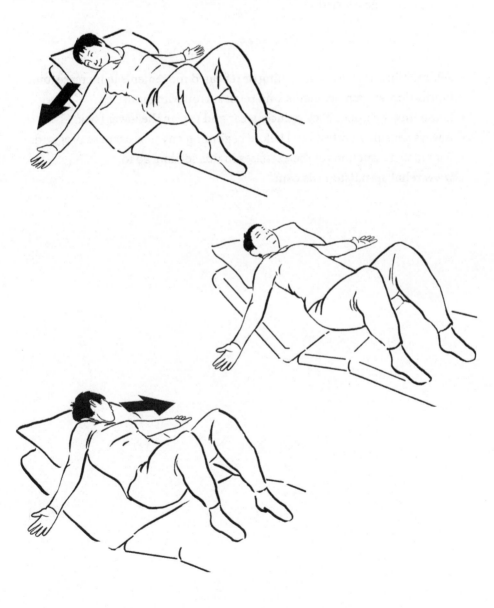

Some people use a foam roller instead of a towel roll. The roller is quite a bit more firm, so I recommend consulting a physical therapist before trying one. Foam rollers can be painful or even injure someone with osteoporosis.

(Notice the emphasis on breathing in this exercise? Deep breathing loosens up the spine and the ribcage. For maximum benefit, make sure you remember to breathe along with the movements.)

Is lying on a towel roll the *only way* to loosen up your upper back? Definitely, not! There are lots of different ways, and different exercises to do this. (Even walking with a pair of trekking poles can help.) I have only chosen the towel roll as an easy place to get started.

SUMMARY

- Self-mobilizations use positioning or repeated movements to increase joint lubrication, stretch ligaments, and relax surrounding muscles.
- Loosening the upper back reduces wear and tear in the lower back.
- Always consult a professional before beginning any new exercise program.
- For video instructions of the exercises in this section, go to **www.rehabspinalstenosis.com**.

KEEP MOVING SUCCESS TIPS

Start Small

Go Slow, Don't Rush

Expect Flare-ups

Avoid Self-Sabotage

Play Music

Use a Checklist

Find a Buddy

Never Punish, Always Reward

Not everyone loves exercise.

In fact, many people h-a-t-e hate it.

I learned this in my first year as a physical therapist when, after eagerly giving a bunch of exercises to my patients, they would come back on their next visit and say, "No, I didn't do them. I just couldn't find the time." It became clear. I could give people exercises till I was blue in the face, but if they didn't *want* to do them, it wasn't going to happen.

This was very shocking news, but after a few days of crying in front of the TV, eating donuts, I moved into the acceptance phase and began trying to figure out how to motivate people to *just do something.*

The following strategies help.

START SMALL

Start small. Very, very small.

Getting started with a new exercise program, sometimes you have to play some tricks on your mind. Your mind says, *I don't have time to go on the treadmill for 30 minutes.* You say, *Well, how about 15?* Your mind says: *I don't even have time for 15 minutes.* You say, *OK, then, two minutes.* Your mind says: *Two minutes isn't going to do anything.* You say: *Two minutes will at least get me onto that treadmill.* So you make a deal with yourself to spend a mere two minutes on the treadmill. After two minutes, guess what happens... You may not want to get OFF the treadmill! Woot! Woot!

You can use this technique for treadmill walking, riding an exercise bike, walking outside (just tell yourself you're walking out to the sidewalk and back), or doing a few reps of a new mat exercise ("I'll just do three of each.").

Starting small is starting smart. Some of you need not only to start small, but stay small. That's OK. Not everyone needs to progress to more advanced exercises. If you are meeting your goals with the easier ones, by all means stick with those.

GO SLOW, DON'T RUSH

Progressing your own exercise program is like playing a game of checkers. It doesn't pay to rush your next move.

Each of the exercises in this book has an infinite number of micro-stages built into it to make it easier or harder. When starting an exercise for the first time, keep movements small. Limit yourself to five or ten reps. I also recommend this one very simple rule:

> *Always wait at least two days after adding a new exercise to see how your body responds.*

If an exercise makes you feel worse, you can either stop doing it completely, or try doing a more basic version with less effort. Sometimes you will need to find a different position to try it in.

Once you know you can do an exercise without flaring yourself up, congratulate yourself. Then, try not to move on too quickly. Doing more reps of an easier exercise gets you ready to try something more difficult.

EXPECT FLARE-UPS

A flare-up is basically a sudden worsening of your symptoms. Flare-ups happen from time to time with all arthritic conditions (spinal stenosis being one of them), and they are sometimes related to some movement or activity and sometimes seemingly random. Even bad weather can set something off.

Anyone with spinal stenosis can have a bad day or week. The main thing is not to panic. Panic and stress can exacerbate pain. You have the tools to manage your symptoms.

DURING A FLARE-UP

- Go back to the chapter on controlling inflammation and follow the instructions.
- Don't stop exercising completely, just go back to your most non-aggravating exercises.
- Try doing your exercises more gently. Reduce your effort level to 25%. If 25% flares you up, go with 10% effort level.

Notify your physician if you have any of the following symptoms: trouble with bowel or bladder control, persistent loss of strength or sensation in your legs, sudden severe low back pain, genital numbness.

USE ICE TO PREVENT FLARE-UPS

We already know ice can reduce inflammation. But ice can also be used to *prevent* inflammation. This means *ice can be used to prevent flare-ups*. Use it after you do a new exercise program. Use it after you go for a walk. Use it not just if you're feeling sore—but even before you're feeling sore. Review the section on decreasing inflammation for safe parameters on using ice.

AVOID SELF-SABOTAGE

Self-sabotage is when your subconscious, for whatever reason, figures out a way for your exercises not to work. The end result is that you throw up your hands and surrender.

Sometimes, I'll give an exercise to someone, and they come back on their next visit with the story of: "Hey, I tried, but I couldn't do that exercise because it hurt me!" Later, I'd find out she went straight to the advanced version or used too much resistance or started (against all advice) with too many repetitions. Why?

"Because I couldn't *feel* it."

Well, what she couldn't feel was the *easier* version of the exercise—which she'd been able to do quite comfortably. This goes back to the whole "start small" thing.

Another form of self-sabotage might be doing a lot of additional activities (going to a museum and standing all day, trimming those rose bushes you've been meaning to get to for months)—on the very same day you add a new exercise, then blaming the exercise for making you sore.

PLAY MUSIC — NO, PLAY YOUR *FAVORITE* MUSIC

Music has such an amazing effect on people! I encountered a patient in the hospital once with both Parkinson's and Alzheimer's disease. "Lawrence" had not walked in months and needed to be lifted into a wheelchair. At patient conference one morning, Lawrence's daughter told me her father had used to love dancing the Charleston. That afternoon, the occupational therapist and I eased Lawrence into a standing position. We began to sing: "Charleston! Charleston! Doo doo doo doo doo doo."

His face lit up! He actually started dancing the Charleston right there. And he was *good* at it. He began to sing along with us, and even let go of my hand to snap his fingers. From then on, instead of trying (and failing) to walk Lawrence down the hall, we *Charlestoned* him down the hall.

If music can have this kind of effect on a man who couldn't get out of bed, what kind of effect might it have on you?

USE A CHECKLIST

Post a checklist on the back of your front door or refrigerator. Check off each day that you do your exercises. Shoot for four or more check marks per week. Remember each check mark brings you closer to your goal.

FIND A BUDDY TO KEEP YOU ACCOUNTABLE

Ask a reliable friend to help keep you on track for your exercise program. Pick a time each day when you're going to do your exercises. Send your buddy a text each time you're about to do them. Your buddy can text you back: "Good job!"

Your buddy can also text you if you don't do your exercises: "Hey, when's a good time to catch up on those exercises you missed this morning? Now?"

NEVER PUNISH, ALWAYS REWARD

Lots of people who hate exercise do so because they see it as a punishment. When they *do* exercise, they often do too much, thinking, *No pain, no gain.* They beat themselves up for being lazy instead of praising themselves for giving it a try. A better way of taking care of yourself is to do one exercise, very few reps, 3–4 times per day. Tell yourself how great you are each time you finish. Go to the mirror, look yourself in the eye, and say, "You are awesome."

YOU ARE AWESOME!

Improve Health and Wellness

< FOCUS AREA 3 >

HEALTHY PEOPLE, BETTER OUTCOMES

Although "Improve Health and Wellness" is the *last* focus area in this section, it is by no means the least important. In fact, most current research suggests the opposite. A recent study out of France found the *only* statistically relevant factor toward a favorable outcome for one type of spinal stenosis surgery was the health and wellness of the patient.

Why is this true? Because healthy people have healthy tissues. When you have the best possible circulation to your discs, bones, nerves, ligaments, and fascia combined with low levels of inflammation and toxicity in your system, you have the best chance for reduced pain and fewer symptoms. You have the best chance to heal, the best chance to be a symptom-free person with spinal stenosis.

Although some health issues are beyond our control, I'm going to discuss some of the ones we can do something about. Whether you're in constant severe pain or have minimal symptoms, the following lifestyle changes will give you the best possible chance of improving your symptoms, with or without surgery.

Smoking. It's one of the hardest things to quit, and one of the worst things you can do for lumbar spinal stenosis. When you light up a cigarette, your capillaries constrict. Those networks of tiny blood vessels carrying nutrients to your tissues? The only blood vessels responsible for the exchange of fluids between cells? Well, they just stop delivering up the goods.

Sorry. Store's closed!

The ends of your toes have very small capillary beds, as do the teeth and gums. But the smallest, scarcest capillary beds—so fragile and delicate, their existence was not even known about until recently—are those that supply nutrients to the discs in your spine. Smoking essentially starves your spine of nutrients, rolling out the welcome mat for early degenerative changes.

Sorry, discs.

Sorry, cartilage.

Sorry, ligaments.

Let's talk about ligaments. Take away their blood supply and these smooth sheets of elastic tissue, intricately layered and functioning to perfection, get all thick and nasty like a bunch of worn out fan belts.

Besides constricting the capillary beds (nicotine is a vasoconstrictor), smoking also fills your blood with carbon monoxide, which essentially poisons the discs, ligaments, and nerves—whatever parts of them the blood can still get to.

My friend Eric specializes in working with hand surgery patients. He says his patients who smoke often have problems with their surgical scars closing. "I tell them, just take two weeks off from smoking and see what happens to your wound. I can't tell you how many times I've convinced someone to do this and when they do, wounds that have refused to heal for months just close right up within about ten days."

Originally, I meant to offer details on quitting smoking, listing all kinds of things to try: the patch, electronic cigarettes, hypnotherapy, self-hypnosis tapes, support groups, acupuncture, Chantix, and so on. But, most smokers have heard about all these. It's really up to the individual to figure out his or her best approach, which is usually a combination of many different strategies to be discussed with a qualified professional.

Health-related perks of non-smoking include:

- Reduction of the risk of developing diabetes.
- Improved lung and cardiac function.
- Improved circulation and number of capillaries.
- Improved chance of being symptom-free with lumbar spinal stenosis.

The good news about quitting smoking? Even after multiple failed attempts, you can still keep trying. In fact, the more times you try to quit, the more likely you are to finally succeed.

Drink More Water, Less Alcohol

Excessive consumption of alcohol (more than one drink per day for women and two drinks per day for men) raises the risk of coronary artery disease, stroke, high blood pressure, cardiac arrhythmias, heart failure, and diabetes. All these problems lead to less circulation to your spine, more disc degeneration and arthritis, and more progression and symptoms of lumbar spinal stenosis.

Conversely, making sure you stay hydrated by drinking plenty of water can benefit spinal stenosis by improving circulation and the health of your discs.

Achieve a Healthy Weight

A person's weight can be an awkward subject. The overweight suffer from discrimination and judgment enough. However, obesity is also a risk factor related to spinal stenosis. It also increases the chances of getting diabetes (80–90% of people diagnosed with type II diabetes are also diagnosed as obese), which reduces the body's ability to heal and contributes to stenosis.

Health-related perks of achieving a healthy weight include:

- Lowered blood pressure.
- Better blood sugar levels.
- Reduced knee pain (which leads to a smoother gait) and improved spinal alignment.
- Higher energy levels.
- Better endurance and lung efficiency with subsequently higher levels of oxygen flowing to your spine.

Always consult your physician before beginning any new exercise or weight loss program.

Get Regular Aerobic Exercise

Aerobic exercise gets your heart pumping a little faster and your lungs working a little harder. Examples include: walking, cycling, rollerblading, and swimming. Health-related perks include:

- improved pain tolerance (thanks to an increase in endorphin levels)
- improved health of the cardiovascular system
- possible reduction in the need to be on diabetes or blood pressure medication*
- reduced symptoms of spinal stenosis

One of the challenges of spinal stenosis is that it can rob you of the ability to engage in the easiest form of aerobic exercise: walking. People just assume, "If I can't walk, I can't exercise." But you could ride a bike, or do some mat exercises, use a rowing machine, or shuttle-walk from one spot to another with frequent sitting breaks in between. Or get out there with some walking sticks--or even a four-wheel walker. The important thing is to keep moving any way you can!

Finding the right aerobic exercise for you takes persistence and, at times, creativity. You may also benefit aerobically from short bursts of exercise, with rest breaks between. For assistance on adding aerobic exercise to your wellness program, please review this book's "Focus Area 2: Keep Moving with Strategic Exercise" and consult a physical therapist or physician.

Improve Nutrition

Processed foods full of sugar, salt, and trans fats are about the yummiest things in the world, if you ask me. But let's face it, they are definitely not good for you! If you eat a lot of fast food, or have a pile of Hostess Donettes wrappers living under the seat of your car (so your spouse won't see), or consider a good dinner to be maybe a whole pint of Ben and Jerry's with some cheese puffs, you have an increased risk for developing diabetes, obesity, and heart disease—conditions associated with lumbar spinal stenosis and degenerative joint disease.

TRANS FATS: *man-made fats that extend the amount of time a product can stay on the shelf — eeyuck!*

*Note: any changes in medication must be in collaboration with your physician.

I've discussed how important it can be to decrease inflammation in your spine. The nutritional aspect of that is to reduce consumption of sugar, including high fructose corn syrup. According to nutritional consultant and researcher Christopher James Clark in his book *Nutritional Grail: Ancestral Wisdom, Breakthrough Science, and the Dawning Nutritional Renaissance*, "Excessive sugar consumption is the common thread connecting most degenerative diseases."

Consult your doctor or a nutritionist for advice on how to adjust your diet based on established nutritional principles. A balanced diet with more fresh vegetables, fruit, whole grains, and protein is a great place to start.

Get Plenty of Sleep

Adequate sleep is a key part of a healthy lifestyle, and can benefit your heart, weight, mind, and more.

Believe it or not, improving your sleep habits can help you:

- **Reduce Inflammation**. People who get less sleep—six or less hours per night— have higher blood levels of inflammatory proteins than those who get more.
- **Improve Physical Performance and Stamina**. One study found that athletes who tried to sleep at least 10 hours a night over the course of 6–8 weeks improved their performance levels in speed and endurance.
- **Achieve a Healthy Weight**. Dieters who are well rested lose more fat than those who are sleep deprived.
- **Reduce Stress**. Sleep reduces stress levels and this improves blood pressure, lowers cholesterol, and reduces heart disease.

Trying to get more sleep isn't always as easy as going to bed early or deciding to sleep in. Sleep apnea (the temporary stopping of breathing during sleep) is an often untreated problem that robs your body of the health benefits of sleep, contributing to **high blood pressure, heart failure, stroke, obesity**, and **heart attack**. Signs of apnea include loud snoring or gasping during sleep, as well as daytime sleepiness.

If you think you may have sleep apnea, check with your physician. You may have to undergo a sleep study, which involves being monitored while you do my favorite activity! If the study confirms that you do have sleep apnea, a CPAP machine just might rock your world. These machines use a slight increase in air pressure to keep your airway open while you sleep. But a CPAP machine is just one treatment option. For some people, dental devices have also been effective. A doctor or sleep specialist may help determine the right choice for you.

Listen to Your Body

Are you the typical Type A personality? Always on the go? Do you put other people's needs ahead of yours? Do you often find yourself thinking or saying (especially to friends or your physical therapist, when they advise you to take it easy), "If I don't do it, it won't get done!" or "If I don't do it, it won't get done *right!*" Do you take on more than you should? Will you help a friend move that heavy piece of furniture even though you know you'll pay for it later?

Listening to your body means *not* trying to push through your symptoms. So many of us have had the whole "no pain, no gain" motto drummed into our psyches. Well, this doesn't really work for spinal stenosis. Learn to say no to stenosis-irritating activities—or learn to plan ahead. You can go to that Renaissance festival or art show—just make sure there are plenty of opportunities to sit down, rest, and take care of yourself.

Meditate

It costs nothing, takes no physical skill, and requires only a few minutes per day. What's not to love about some good old-fashioned meditation? According to an article in "Scientific American" (November, 2014), meditation is like the ideal drug. There's evidence that the practice's ability to improve wellbeing can help decrease inflammation and other "biological stresses that occur at the molecular level."

> *Feelings come and go like clouds in a windy sky.*
> *Conscious breathing is my anchor.*
>
> —Thich Nhat Hanh, *Stepping into Freedom:*
> *Rules of Monastic Practice for Novices*

If you're not sure how to meditate, there are a number of good books (and even some excellent YouTube videos) out there that can help. Jennifer Brooks's *The Meditation Transformation: How to Relax and Revitalize Your Body, Your Work, and Your Perspective Today* is a great beginner's starting point. I also recommend Pema Chödrön's *How to Meditate: A Practical Guide to Making Friends with Your Mind* as an enjoyable read with a little humor. You might also purchase (or download one of the many available free) guided meditations. Then all you have to do is find a comfortable spot to relax while you listen and just let yourself...drift.

Planning on icing your back for ten minutes? Why not do a little meditation while you chill out?

SUMMARY

The presence of co-morbidities (high blood pressure, diabetes, obesity, heart disease) is directly related to the degree of symptoms in spinal stenosis patients, both non-surgical and surgical. Tackling any of the above wellness suggestions improves your overall health and contributes to the reduction of spinal stenosis symptoms.

The previously-listed suggestions are interrelated. Becoming a non-smoker, achieving a healthy weight, improving nutrition, and getting regular aerobic exercise all decrease your risk of developing diabetes and improve your cardiac health. Your best bet for success may be to pick one thing to focus on at a time. Once you achieve a positive change, move on to another.

Best of luck!

KEY POINTS

- Your health and wellness level affects your spinal stenosis.
- People with a lower number of health problems have better outcomes after spinal stenosis surgery.
- Making one single wellness change can improve your overall health in many different ways.
- Health and wellness are affected by stress.

SAFETY REVIEW

- Always consult your physician before beginning any new exercise, nutritional, or weight loss program.
- A physician can refer you to a qualified dietician or nutritionist to help you customize a plan.
- You do not need to consult a physician before attempting to meditate. (Just saying.)

PART THREE

Surgery

Some physical therapists have an "avoid surgery at all costs" philosophy. I'm not one of those. Maybe this comes from working with many excellent surgeons, but the bottom line for me is this: Sometimes surgery is in the best interest of the patient. For those of you for whom this is true (or in case you're just curious), I've included this short section discussing surgery for lumbar stenosis.

In my introduction, I presented four individuals: Bud, Lorraine, Yukio, and Sylvia. All of them had severe spinal stenosis according to their MRIs, but none of them wound up needing surgery. Why did I use them as examples? To illustrate that you CAN have *severe spinal stenosis* and NOT have *severe symptoms*.

I wanted to give you a sense of optimism because, in my experience, pessimism is something that is not so good for healing. So many times I have had to talk someone down—someone with very minimal symptoms—because they read their horrible MRI report, saw words like "degenerative" and "disc herniation" and decided right then that there was no hope. How were they supposed to know degenerative changes are found in up to 70% of people who don't have any symptoms? Or that herniated discs are found in up to 50% of people who—you guessed it— don't have any pain.

Back to our four friends with severe spinal stenosis. Did these individuals have severe pain? Yes, but the pain went away fairly quickly with a little bit of icing and some exercise. None of them had severe neurological problems. No loss of control of bowel or bladder function. No numbness in the genital region. No drop foot, progressive weakness, or constant numbness and tingling. This is more important and indicative of whether a person needs surgery.

Now, are you *more likely* to have mild symptoms when you have milder spinal stenosis? Yes, but you are not *guaranteed* to have milder symptoms than your neighbor who has severe stenosis. The severity of your symptoms—not the MRI result—is what primarily dictates the necessity for surgery.

Generally speaking, a doctor's first choice of treatment for patients *without* severe symptoms (regardless of the severity of their MRI result!) is what is called "conservative treatment" or "medical/interventional care." This basically includes things such as:

- Medication (oral anti-inflammatory medication)
- Epidural Injections (anti-inflammatory medication injected into the affected area of the spine)
- Physical Therapy (exercise, self-management education, and modalities)
- Acupuncture
- Other Alternative Non-Surgical Treatments
- Just Playing the Waiting Game (Hey, don't laugh--it has a 50% success rate!)

Keep in mind that when I use the term "severe symptoms," I am not including severe pain in that category, because severe pain can often get better very quickly without surgery. Hence, you can be in very severe pain, and still learn that your doctor's first recommendation for treatment is "conservative" or "non-surgical." Believe me, this is no reason for you to feel ripped off.

This brings us to the person who *would be* a candidate for surgery. This person would be:

- A person with severe neurological deficits that require an emergency surgery to prevent further or rapid deterioration or permanent nerve damage.
- A person who has failed to improve with the previous listed "non-surgical" treatments and whose quality of life is such that he or she feels the risks of surgery are outweighed by the potential benefits.

In addition to the above, your spine surgeon must deem you to be a "good surgical candidate" based on certain criteria that indicate a good chance for a positive outcome.

SO WHAT MAKES ME A GOOD SURGICAL CANDIDATE?

Spine surgeons hold themselves to a very tough standard—selecting patients for surgery who meet certain standardized criteria. Some (not all) of these are listed below:

- *The patient's stenosis is causing severe neurological problems.*
  (progressive weakness, stumbling, drop foot, loss of bowel or bladder control)
- *The patient has gotten no relief from non-surgical interventions.*
  (medication, injections, physical therapy)
- *The patient has a low number of "co-morbidities."*
  (smoking, advanced age, obesity, depression, diabetes, heart disease)
- *The MRI or CT scan shows significant impingement of the spinal canal or nerve roots.*
  (matching the same area of nerve deficit or pain in the patient)

Guidelines for choosing surgery may be standardized, but there will still be differences of opinion between surgeons as to whether you are a good candidate. Some surgeons will not do surgery on anyone who smokes. Others may require you to make certain wellness changes for a period of time before surgery.

SURGICAL TERMS

Most lumbar stenosis patients who need surgery will have what's called a "spinal decompression." This is just a general term for various ways to relieve pressure on the spinal canal and nerves. I've listed some common surgical terms related to spinal stenosis below. Looking this over before talking about surgery with your doctor may help keep you from drowning in a sea of medical terminology.

- *Spinal Decompression Surgery*—a general term for the various surgeries that can relieve pressure on the spinal cord and nerve roots. This is the typical surgery for lumbar spinal stenosis.

- *Discectomy*—surgeon takes out all or part of a disc.

- *Microdiscectomy*—surgeon uses a small incision and a long metal tube to take out part of a disc.

- *Laminectomy*—surgeon takes out a portion of the spine bone called the lamina. The lamina is the part of the bone positioned behind the spinal cord. If you were lying on your stomach and your spine bone was a little crock pot or something like that, the laminectomy would be the surgeon just removing the lid to the pot. What protects the spinal cord once that part of the bone is gone? Various layers of back muscles, thank goodness!

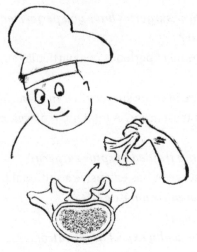

[ARTWORK BY T. NIGHT]

- *Laminotomy*—less drastic than a laminectomy because the surgeon only takes out a little section of the lid to your crockpot.

- *Foraminotomy*—essentially, a "Roto-Rooter" type of job on a nerve opening or openings.

- *Spinal Fusion*—after decompression, metal rods and screws are used to fix together one or more spine bones. This is most often used when more than one level (example: L3–L5) is affected. A fusion may also be necessary if you have *spondylolisthesis* (see page 27) or instability in your spine.

- *Minimally Invasive Technique*—uses smaller incisions and tiny scopes. Similar to an arthroscopic knee surgery. Advantages: faster healing, less disruptive to tissue, and lower rates of infection. Includes *microdiscectomy* and *microdecompression*. Disadvantages: expensive, may not be readily available to your surgeon, and not right for every surgery.

- *Microdecompression Surgery*— decompression of the spinal cord and nerves using minimally invasive techniques

WHO DOES SPINE SURGERY?

Spine surgeries are generally performed by either an orthopedic surgeon or a neurosurgeon.

QUESTIONS TO ASK YOUR SURGEON

As a patient, you have a right to ask some basic questions when interviewing a potential spine surgeon, such as:

- *How many of these surgeries have you performed? How many do you perform per year?*
  Surgeons with more experience in a particular surgery often have better results.
- *Do you specialize in spine surgery? Or in a specific type of spine surgery?*
  Who would you trust more? A total hip replacement specialist? Or a spine specialist?
  Are you fellowship trained in spine surgery?
  Indicates your surgeon has extensive additional training in spine surgery.
- *What is your complication rate?*
  Is it above the norm?
- *What can I realistically expect as an outcome?*
  Include letting the surgeon know what your expectations are, and getting those clarified before you have surgery.
- *What kind of surgery are you going to do?*
  You should understand the procedure to the extent that you are interested. Some people, I understand, just don't want to know. But if your doctor isn't willing to take the time to explain....

REALISTIC OUTCOMES AND EXPECTATIONS

Occasionally, I meet a client who tells me the story of how he confronted his surgeon with the following question: "Can you absolutely guarantee me this will fix my problem?" When the poor surgeon answers, "Of course, not," the patient replies, "Well, then I'm not doing it!"

While expecting a guarantee from a surgeon is completely unrealistic, if you do need surgery for stenosis, you have reasons to be optimistic. (And optimism is good for you! It actually promotes healing!) According to a 2008 article in *The New England Journal of Medicine*, "80% of patients have some degree of symptomatic relief after surgery for spinal stenosis."

RECOVERING FROM SURGERY

In addition to working with private clients, and clients in outpatient clinics, I've been fortunate enough to extend my practice to the field of home health. Over the past six years, I've been visiting people at home during those first crucial weeks immediately after spine surgery. These are a few things I've found helpful to remember.

It is important to make sure your pain is under control. If your pain is not well-controlled, you will be tense. And if you are tense, your back muscles will be tense. And this will make you feel worse. This means taking your pain medication as prescribed, not waiting for your pain to become excruciating. It also means communicating with your doctor if, when taking your medication as prescribed, your pain does become excruciating.

Breathing exercises can help you relax. And relaxation (as opposed to worrying) is beneficial to healing.

Pain medication can constipate you. Take your stool softener, drink your prune juice, take the advice of your home health nurse, and so on. Don't ignore constipation for days.

Some people have numbness, tingling, or weakness in their leg or legs right after surgery. While this is something you should notify your doctor about, these types of symptoms often improve over time.

Your surgeon's office may give you some materials to read, instructions on how to care for your incision, how to get in and out of bed, how much you can safely lift, and so on. Follow those instructions for best results after surgery.

Do not, in your first year after surgery, help your friend move his refrigerator, piano, or sofa. Just my opinion, for what it's worth. You'd be surprised how many people do this.

SUMMARY

Many people with lumbar spinal stenosis can improve over time without surgery. However, if it turns out that--either because of neurological problems or intolerable quality of life--you do need surgery, you have reasons to be optimistic. And you can still use the strategies from the following three focus areas:

- Reduce Inflammation
- Keep Moving with Strategic Exercise
- Improve Health and Wellness

These strategies are designed to help you reach your best possible outcome.

KEY POINTS

- A person can have severe spinal stenosis *with or without* severe symptoms.
- A person can have only mild spinal stenosis *with or without* severe symptoms.
- The severity of your symptoms is an important factor in determining if you need surgery.
- Severe pain that goes away in a week or two with good self-management is not usually an indication for surgery.
- The recommended first choice of treatment in a patient having stenosis, but without severe symptoms, is "conservative treatment" or "medical interventional care."
- Prior to performing surgery, some surgeons may ask you to quit smoking or make other wellness changes, such as getting your blood sugar under control.
- It's a good idea to interview your surgeon and ask about success rates.

APPENDIX

25 Tips for
Lumbar Spinal Stenosis

1. ***Ride an exercise bike.*** Work out while decreasing pressure on the spinal cord and nerves. A great alternative to walking.

2. ***Stop forcing yourself to stand up straight.*** If you're comfortable standing up straight, great. But if standing up straight is making your legs feel rubbery or your low back feel like it's going to cave in, you're better off finding a nice place to sit down.

3. ***Use an elastic lumbar corset.*** Helps limit large movements. Helps if you're going to be on your feet a little longer than usual. Wear it while you sleep to reduce awful morning wake-up pain.

4. ***Use ice.*** Slows down the nerve's ability to conduct pain signals and increases circulation to your spine. Ice also causes deep muscle relaxation.

5. ***Use a walker with a seat.*** A walker with fold-down seat lets you sit down whenever you need to and is great for preventing falls. Especially useful if you have trouble walking or standing for long periods.

6. ***Use a Nu-Step machine.*** It lets you sit while you exercise

7. ***Share this book with friends and family.*** You need them to understand what you're going through. (And to stop nagging you to "stand up straight")

8. ***Buy a recliner.*** Recliners let you rest in a comfortably flexed position. Just remember to get out of it and move around frequently.

9. ***Lie down (or recline) and strengthen your legs.*** Do more repetitions (because you're not standing) and experience less fatigue (because you're not standing) exercising in a position in which your nerves are firing full-cylinder.

10. ***Get regular aerobic exercise.*** Increases the general health of all tissues. Aerobic exercise is the single most important factor in whether an individual has back pain.

11. ***Do Breathing Exercises.*** Studies show a strong connection between breathing disorders and back pain.

12. ***Do Tai Chi.*** This type of moving meditation has a number of health benefits. Tai Chi reduces stress levels, improves circulation, and strengthens deep muscles that provide support and enhance blood flow to the spine.

13. **Try acupuncture.** Increases the general health of all tissues, including circulation and metabolism.

14. **Stop smoking.** If aerobic exercise increases the general health of all tissues, smoking decreases the general health of all tissues. It particularly reduces circulation of the capillary beds, the smallest of which just happen to reside in the intervertebral discs.

15. **Get your blood sugar under control.** Out of control blood sugar means out-of-control ligaments, as in ligamentous thickening and pain.

16. **Exercise muscles that connect to the deepest parts of your spine,** including the *tranverse abdominus* muscle and *latissimus dorsi* (or "lats").

17. **Avoid sit ups, crunches, leg lifts, and any other zany exercises that torque your spine or pelvis.** These types of exercises are great for making you feel like crap. (Exception: you are already doing these types of exercises and they make you feel great!)

18. **Avoid extreme rotational exercises.** Especially if you have foraminal stenosis, lying down and dropping your knees from side to side can be the equivalent of pinching your nerves over and over with a pair of pliers.

19. **Get your upper back moving.** The more flexible your upper back and rib cage, the less pressure on your lower back. Use the exercises and positioning techniques provided in this book to create movement in your thoracic spine.

20. **Use a kitchen stool.** Like to cook? Take breaks from prolonged standing on your beautiful new kitchen stool.

21. **Reduce your alcohol consumption.** Fits into the same category as "stop smoking" and "control your blood sugar." It's all about circulation, improved tissue nutrition, metabolism, and health.

22. **Get a hot tub.** Just because.

23. **Consult a spine surgeon.** Do this immediately if you have any loss of bowel or bladder control, numbness in the genital region, or if the weakness in your legs is severe. Many surgeons prefer a conservative approach with people whose symptoms are not severe, and they can be a resource for other types of treatment such as anti-inflammatory medications, injections, or even a good physical therapist, chiropractor, or acupuncturist.

24. **Adjust your computer station.** Because stiffness in the upper back can wreak havoc with your lower back.

25. **Listen to your body.** Learn to give yourself breaks. Pushing through the pain does not work for spinal stenosis.

Glossary of Terms

Capillaries: the tiniest blood vessels, and the only blood vessels whose walls permit the exchange of blood and fluids with surrounding cells and tissue. Essential for microcirculation—and hence for the health of ligaments, muscles, bones and discs.

Cauda Equina: though it sounds like some villain from a Shakespearean play, the *cauda equina* (Latin for "horse's tail") is actually a bundle of spinal nerves running through the lower half of your spinal cord canal. These nerves exit the lumbar spine at its lowest levels and are responsible for signals to the hips, knees, ankles, feet, anal sphincter, and bladder.

Co-morbidities: One disease or health issue, that's a *morbidity*. A bunch of different diseases or health issues, those are *co-morbidities*. Much like when you have a bunch of annoying pathological personalities in a co-operative living situation, a bunch of annoying pathological co-morbidities will play off each other and multiply your health problems.

Compression fracture: the collapse of a vertebra. Often associated with osteoporosis and aging. Compression fractures make your spine bones shaped like little triangles instead of little cubes.

Dura Mater: (derived from the Latin for *tough mother*) a thick, leather-like membrane that surrounds and protects the spinal cord. Also known as "the Dura."

Epidural Space: the space inside the spinal canal. Basically, everything outside the *dura*, but inside the donut-hole sized tunnel that runs through your spine. Also known as the *cord space*.

Facet joints: Tiny joints in your spine connecting one spine bone to another. When you twist, your facets open and close like tiny fish mouths. These joints can develop spurs (osteophytes) and thickened ligaments. When this happens, they can eventually fuse. Then twisting isn't as much fun anymore.

Fascia: A beautiful substance, with the ability to both expand and contract, fascia is this moist, elastic cobwebby stuff that permeates our bodies and basically connects...well, just everything.

Foramina: these are the little ear-shaped holes the nerves travel through and out of on either side of your spine; one is called a *foramen*. Sometimes, your doctor will tell you have *foraminal narrowing,* which just means there isn't a lot of space for your nerve.

Fusion: the loss of a joint's ability to move. Associated with loss of movement, circulation, and degenerative arthritis.

Intervertebral Discs: round cushions acting both as shock absorbers and spacers between the spine bones. The more space created between two spine bones, the easier and better the movement. Discs become less hydrated and flatter as we age. Also known as the *intervertebral fibrocartilage*, these cushions have a very small capillary system and can easily miss out on essential nutrients and hydration.

Intervertebral Foramina: hole through which a nerve root exits the spine.

Ischemia: lack of blood supply to any tissue. Ischemia can lead to swelling, death of tissue, loss of elasticity.

Ligament: Tissue that connects bones to other bones. Healthy ligaments are elastic, lengthening under tension, and returning to their original shape when tension is removed. Ligaments that lose their elasticity are like old rubber bands put on slack. They just wad up—not doing their job and taking up space. You have two major ligaments in the spinal canal—one type in front and another type in the back. Both take up more than their fair share of space when they lose their healthy elastic state of being.

Ligamenta Flava (yellow ligaments): these ligaments made of yellowish fibro-elastic tissue live behind the spinal cord at the back of the spinal canal. They help you stand up straight, including helping you straighten while getting up from a chair. When you're standing, the marked *elasticity* of these ligaments (when healthy) prevents them from buckling into the *spinal canal*. Thickening of these ligaments, along with a loss of elasticity, makes them take up space in the spinal canal. In extreme cases, they can simply turn right into bone. You have a bunch of these. Each one is called a ligamentum flavum. That's how Latin folks do the whole singular and plural thing.

Ligamentum Flavum hypertrophy: thickening of the ligamentum flavum (equals less space for the spinal cord).

Neurogenic Claudication: a fancy name for the annoying weakness, numbness, and cramping in the buttocks, thighs, and calves related to being on your feet for too long. (Not to be confused with vascular claudication—a similar type of problem caused by poor circulation in the legs.) The word claudication comes from the Latin claudicare, which means "to limp." Neurogenic claudication is the chief symptom of central lumbar spinal stenosis.

Osteophytes: bony spurs that form along the edges of bones. Found in 90% of men over 50 and 90% of women over 60.

Posterior Longitudinal Ligament (PLL): This long ligament runs from the very top of your neck all the way to your tailbone and is positioned in the front part of the spinal canal (behind the intervertebral discs). The PLL is inherently attached to the back part of each of your discs. Much like the ligamentum flavum, thickening of the PLL takes up much needed space in the spinal cord canal and contributes to spinal stenosis.

Pre-symptomatic Walking Distance (PSWD): the distance a person can walk before the onset of symptoms.

Pre-symptomatic Walking Time (PSWT): the amount of time a person can walk before the onset of symptoms.

Sacralization: when the very last vertebra in your low back begins to fuse with the sacrum.

Spinal Canal: the hole running down the center of your spine, through which the spinal cord travels. Narrowing of the spinal canal is called central canal stenosis.

Spondylolisthesis: basically, the forward slipping of a bone in your spine. Usually happens at the very base of the spine, or the 5th lumbar vertebra. This slippage creates less room in the spinal canal.

Vertebra: a single bone in your spine; changes shape as you age and can develop bony calluses in the form of lipping and spurring.

Vertebrae: more than one spine bone; no big whoop.

Bibliography

Barker PJ, Briggs CA, Bogeski G, "Tensile transmission across the lumbar fasciae in unembalmed cadavers: effects of tension to various muscular attachments." *Spine* (Phila Pa 1976). 2004 January.

Barker PJ, Urquhart DM, Story IH, Fahrer M, Briggs CA, "The middle layer of lumbar fascia and attachments to lumbar transverse processes: implications for segmental control and fracture." *European Spine Journal.* 2007 December.

Bogduk N, Johnson G, Spalding D, "The morphology and biomechanics of latissimus dorsi." *Clinical Biomechanics.* (Bristol, Avon) 1998 September.

Gatton ML, Pearcy MJ, Pettet GJ, Evans JH, "A three-dimensional mathematical model of the thoracolumbar fascia and an estimate of its biomechanical effect." *Journal of Biomechanics.* 2010 October.

Gunzburg R, Szpalski M (editors), *Lumbar Spinal Stenosis.* (Lippincott Williams & Wilkins) 2000.

Halet KA, Mayhew JL, Murphy C, Fanthorpe J, "Relationship of 1 repetition maximum lat-pull to pull-up and lat-pull repetitions in elite collegiate women swimmers." *J The Journal of Strength and Conditioning Research.* 2009 August.

Hartjen CA, Resnick DK, Hsu KY, Zucherman JF, Hsu EH, Skidmore GA, "Two-Year Evaluation of the X-STOP Interspinous Spacer in Different Primary Patient Populations With Neurogenic Intermittent Claudication due to Lumbar Spinal Stenosis." *Journal of Spinal Disorders and Techniques.* 2012 November.

Hocking DC, Titus PA, Sumagin R, Sarelius IH, "Extracellular matrix fibronectin mechanically couples skeletal muscle contraction with local vasodilation." *Circulation Research.* 2008 Feb 15.

Hur JW, Hur JK, Kwon TH, Park YK, Chung HS, Kim JH, "Radiological significance of ligamentum flavum hypertrophy in the occurrence of redundant nerve roots of central lumbar spinal stenosis." *Journal of Korean Neurosurgical Society.* 2012 September.

Issack PS, Cunningham ME, Pumberger M, Hughes AP, Cammisa FP Jr, "Degenerative lumbar spinal stenosis: evaluation and management." *Journal of the American Academy of Orthopedic Surgeons.* 2012, August.

Jarrett MS, Orlando JF, Grimmer-Somers K, "The effectiveness of land based exercise compared to decompressive surgery in the management of lumbar spinal-canal stenosis: a systematic review." *BMC Musculoskeletal Disorders.* 2012 February.

Jemmett RS, Macdonald DA, Agur AM, "Anatomical relationships between selected segmental muscles of the lumbar spine in the context of multi-planar segmental motion: a preliminary investigation." *Manual Therapy.* 2004 November.

Kääriäinen T, Leinonen V, Taimela S, Aalto T, Kröger H, Herno A, Turunen V, Savolainen S, Kankaanpää M, Airaksinen O, "Lumbar paraspinal and biceps brachii muscle function and movement perception in lumbar spinal stenosis." *European Spine Journal.* 2012 Nov 21.

Kosaka H, Sairyo K, Biyani A, Leaman D, Yeasting R, Higashino K, Sakai T, Katoh S, Sano T, Goel VK, Yasui N, "Pathomechanism of loss of elasticity and hypertrophy of lumbar ligamentum flavum in elderly patients with lumbar spinal canal stenosis." *Spine.* 2007 December.

Kreiner D. Scott, Baisden J, Gilbert T, Summers J, Toton J, Hwang S, Mendel R, Reitman C, "Diagnosis and Treatment of Degenerative Lumbar Spinal Stenosis." *North American Spine Society: Evidence-Based Clinical Guidelines for Multidisciplinary Spine Care,* 2011.

Kumka M, Bonar J, "Fascia: a morphological description and classification system based on a literature review." *The Journal of the Canadian Chiropractic Association.* 2012 September.

Lorig K, Halsted H, Sobel D, Laurent D, González V, Minor M, *Living a Healthy Life with Chronic Conditions: self-management of heart disease, arthritis, diabetes, depression, asthma, bronchitis, emphysema, and other physical and mental health conditions, Fourth Edition,* (Bull Publishing Company, Boulder, CO), 2012.

Loukas M, Shoja MM, Thurston T, Jones VL, Linganna S, Tubbs RS, "Anatomy and biomechanics of the vertebral aponeurosis part of the posterior layer of the thoracolumbar fascia." *Surgical and Radiologic Anatomy.* 2008 March.

MacDonald DA, Moseley GL, Hodges PW, "The lumbar multifidus: does the evidence support clinical beliefs?" *Manual Therapy.* 2006 November.

May S, Comer C, "Is surgery more effective than non-surgical treatment for spinal stenosis, and which non-surgical treatment is more effective? A systematic review." *Physiotherapy*. 2012 Apr 16.

Rodgers WB, Lehmen JA, Gerber EJ, Rodgers JA, "Grade 2 spondylolisthesis at L4–5 treated by XLIF: safety and midterm results in the "worst case scenario." *Scientific World Journal*. 2012.

Sandella DE, Haig AJ, Tomkins-Lane C, Yamakawa KS, "Defining the Clinical Syndrome of Lumbar Spinal Stenosis: A Recursive Specialist Survey Process." *Physical Medicine and Rehabilitation*. 2012 November.

Sarno, John E, *Healing Back Pain: The Mind-Body Connection*. (Warner Books, Hachette Book Group, New York, NY. 1991.

Schleip R, Klingler W, Lehmann-Horn F, "Active fascial contractility: Fascia may be able to contract in a smooth muscle-like manner and thereby influence musculoskeletal dynamics." *Medical Hypotheses*. 2005.

Starshinov DV, Khodasevich LS, "The influence of physical training on the state of microcirculation in the patients presenting with arterial hypertension when staying at a health resort." *Vopr Kurortol Fizioter Lech Fiz Kult*. 2012 Jan–Feb.

Szpalski M, Gunzburg R, "Lumbar spinal stenosis in the elderly: an overview." *European Spine Journal*. 2003 October.

Willard FH, Vleeming A, Schuenke MD, Danneels L, Schleip R, "The thoracolumbar fascia: anatomy, function and clinical considerations." *Journal of Anatomy*. 2012 December.

Yuan PS, Booth RE Jr, Albert TJ, "Nonsurgical and surgical management of lumbar spinal stenosis." Instructional Course Lecture. 2005.

Zhong ZM, Zha DS, Xiao WD, Wu SH, Wu Q, Zhang Y, Liu FQ, Chen JT, "Hypertrophy of ligamentum flavum in lumbar spine stenosis associated with the increased expression of connective tissue growth factor." *Journal of Orthopedic Research*. 2011 October 29.

Acknowledgments

I would love to thank the following grammatically meticulous individuals, who provided their amazing edits: Lonnie Hull-DuPont, who read the first draft; Elizabeth VanderVen, Michelle Sawyer, my dear Aunt Rose, and Brando Lakes. The keen physical therapist's eye of Noel Tenoso kept me on track with my facts. Davina Kotulski was the perfect writing coach to help me finally get this thing finished!

Much appreciation goes to my talented and tireless illustrator, Tim McGee, who agreed to my many requests for additions, revisions, and coffee dates. John (Hubbard) of Finland, I could not have asked for a more fantastic book design. Various heroic types modeled for the illustrations: David, Shirin, Brando, Paul. A big shout-out goes to a true supermodel, Amanda Han, for doing a whole Sunday's worth of exercises for the videos. Steve Grant did a fantastic job shooting the exercise videos for my web site—wrapping it all up just in time to watch the Seahawks upset the Packers. Oh, yeah.

I am lucky to have the kind of friends who will tell me it's perfectly OK to want to do a "kind of corny healthcare book." Thank you so much for being there Robert Cooper and Tim Welberry, Michelle and Robert Stern, Rose Fabris, Jill Moynahan, Kenna Brinkman, Sharon Kelly, Alberta Zajack, and Jean Amato.

Three cheers to Seattle's Dr. Alexis Falicov for providing a spine surgeon's perspective.

Thanks to Meryl Needles, Sleep Apnea Specialist, for teaching me about sleep apnea and wellness.

To all the colleagues who have supported me and put up with my various ramblings on stenosis, thank you so much.

I would also like to bow down to my clients—especially the tough ones— who, over the years, taught me everything I know, yet kept me aware of how much I didn't—and still don't.

My wife, Elliott Night, has been my support, editor, best critic, and lifeline— not only for this project, but for life.

How nice is that?